THE REFLEXOLOGY WORKOUT

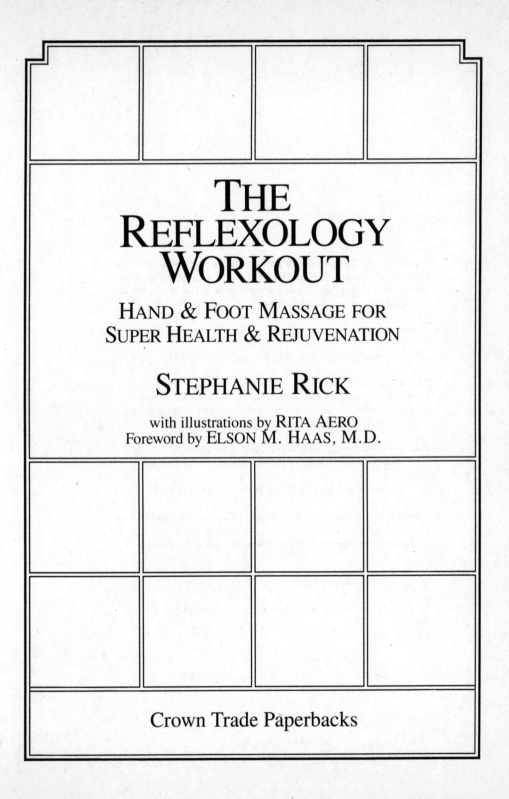

THE REFLEXOLOGY WORKOUT

HAND & FOOT MASSAGE FOR SUPER HEALTH & REJUVENATION

STEPHANIE RICK

with illustrations by RITA AERO
Foreword by ELSON M. HAAS, M.D.

Crown Trade Paperbacks

Publisher's Note: This book includes therapeutic massage instructions and programs for the reader to follow. However, not all massage therapies are designed for all individuals. Before starting these or any other massage or exercise programs you should consult your doctor for advice.

Published by Crown Trade Paperbacks, 201 East 50th Street, New York, New York 10022. Member of the Crown Publishing Group

Previously published by Crown Trade Paperbacks in 1986.

Random House, Inc. New York, Toronto, London, Sydney, Auckland

Crown Trade Paperbacks and colophon are trademarks of Crown Publishers, Inc.

Manufactured in the United States of America

Library of Congress Cataloging-in-Publication Data

Rick, Stephanie
    1. Massage. 2 Reflexotherapy, 3. Hand 4. Foot
    1. Aero, Rita II. Title
    RA780,5.R53   1986   646.7'5   82-31724
    ISBN 0-517-88485-2

10 9 8 7 6 5 4 3 2 1

Second Paperback Edition

CONTENTS

CHARTS OF THE REFLEXES

FOREWORD

by Elson M. Haas, M.D.

Director of the Marin Clinic of Preventive Medicine and Health Education
San Rafael, California

I am very excited to be involved with *The Reflexology Workout* because I believe that it introduces a new depth to this body therapy. In my medical practice, I have incorporated and studied the results of various body therapies, including reflexology. The hands and feet are very sensitive areas, and massaging them through reflexology can refine our body-awareness as we physically experience our internal interconnections. Although reflexology is not an exact science, I find that it releases tension and helps to heal the body through mechanisms not yet completely understood.

This book provides practical and simple-to-use methods for applying reflexology, without suggesting that it can replace traditional medical practices — a pitfall for many new-age health books. It teaches us about our body through basic anatomy and physiology and gives us a clear picture of healthy, functioning organs. When we hold in our mind a positive image of the benefits we will receive from any action, we increase our chances for success. In addition, I found the "Workout" and "Troubleshooting" sections inspiring — offering new ways to enhance the functioning capacity of the body through reflexology treatment.

Reflexology is an ancient and noninvasive therapy. One of the greatest aspects of this system is that it can easily become a helpful self-care technique that can bring healing therapies into the home. Reflexology is personally fulfilling for those of us who practice it, whether on ourselves or in helping others; and it can be applied by family members and friends without fear of injury.

Today, reflexology is in widespread use among medical professionals and healing practitioners. The body's bioenergetic flow — the harmonious alignment of bodily functions and nervous energy — is a prerequisite to good health; and reflexology allows us to experience the internal relationship between our body and our physical and emotional environment. I am optimistic that the benefits that you, the reader, will derive from *The Reflexology Workout* can have a positive influence on the health and vitality of your life.

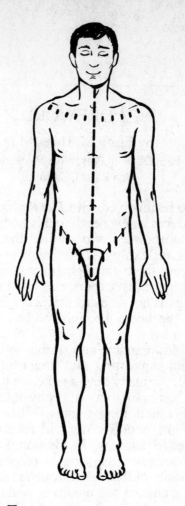

INTRODUCTION

There has been a growing realization, over the past twenty years, that a long and healthy life is not just something that happens to a lucky few, but something that anyone with a commitment to health can achieve. The potential for super health comes through knowledge and self-awareness, through understanding the body and its functions and learning how to control them.

In recent years, the holistic health movement has demystified and brought into modern use many ancient, time-tested methods that humans have used to heal themselves, to prevent disease, and to improve the quality of their lives. Along with acupuncture and herbology, reflexology is receiving renewed attention and is being increasingly integrated into current medical practices.

In Europe today, more than six thousand doctors, nurses, and physical therapists incorporate reflexology into their healing procedures. It is used on patients to relieve their painful sensations, to instill feelings of relaxation, and to speed their healing. As part of their treatment, patients are encouraged to visualize the parts of their body being stimulated by reflexology in order to gain an understanding and sense of control over their physical health.

It is not clear why or how reflexology works — it simply does. A relationship between areas on the hands and feet and the body's organs, limbs, and nerves has been recognized for thousands of years by many civilizations. At the beginning of this century, Dr. William Fitzgerald, an American physician, studied these relationships. Through experimentation, he found that there were specific interactions between areas on the hands and feet and the organs of the body, and that, by pressing these areas, he could directly affect the organs. After further study, he realized that these interactions followed a simple pattern.

Fitzgerald divided the body into ten longitudinal zones, five on each side of the body's midline. Each zone is unique and each has a self-contained environment — every part of the body within that zone interacts with every other part in that zone. Because all the zones are represented on the hands and feet, it became clear to Fitzgerald that they were the most convenient terminals for communicating with the rest of the body. For example, the inner edges of the feet are in the same zone as the spine, so stimulating the inner edges of the feet will then stimulate the spine as well.

The body continuously strives to maintain a delicate metabolic equilibrium, but when this balance is disturbed by injury, disease, or the stress of daily life, it upsets the normal functions of the body, putting its health in jeopardy. Reflexology is a simple and noninvasive method for realigning these functions in order to help the body attain the perfect metabolic balance that leads to super health.

Reflexology and its techniques are presented in this book along with straightforward descriptions of the body and its functions. These will help you understand and visualize what is happening in your body. After you review these, you will want to try the eight reflexology workouts, which are designed to influence your body's metabolic processes in very specific and beneficial ways. The workouts take only minutes to perform and yield remarkable and pleasurable results. If you have specific physical concerns, you will find troubleshooting techniques throughout the book to help you deal with them. Whatever your reasons for exploring reflexology, you are going to discover that it will enhance every facet of your physical health and emotional well-being.

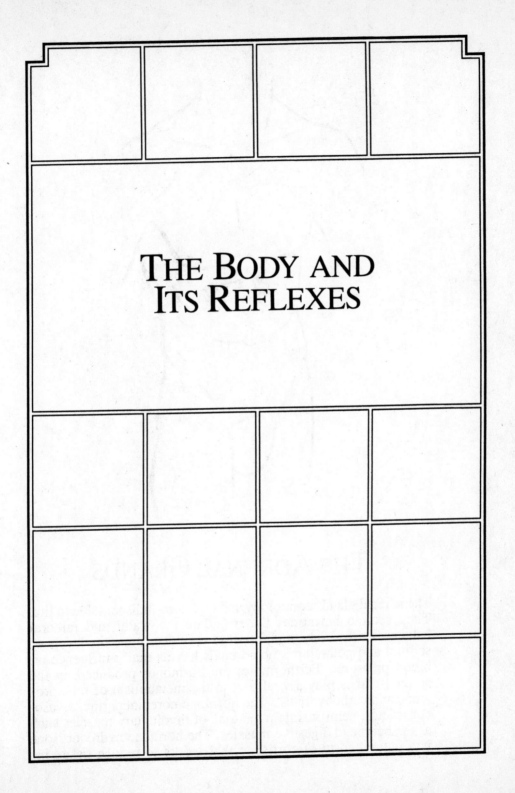

THE BODY AND
ITS REFLEXES

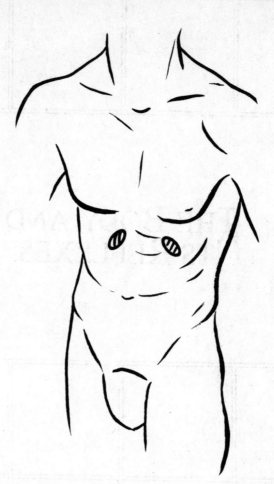

THE ADRENAL GLANDS

The adrenal glands control myriad functions indispensable to life. They secrete hormones that regulate the water and mineral balances in the body, and, because they determine the levels of sodium and potassium, the adrenals have a major influence on blood pressure. Furthermore, the hormones produced by the adrenal glands play a vital part in the metabolism of fats, proteins, and carbohydrates. The hormone norepinephrine, a vasoconstrictor, helps maintain the tone of involuntary muscles such as the heart and digestive muscles. The hormone hydrocortisone is a natural form of cortisone that works to reduce tissue inflammation. Another hormone, commonly known by its trade name Adrenalin, is epinephrine, which serves as the body's front-line defense against fatigue.

When confronted with an emergency situation, most people display a "fight-or-flight" reaction. The adrenal glands receive a signal from the sympathetic nervous system to release epinephrine. This hormone triggers the release of glucose for a quick burst of energy and stimulates the heart, increasing the blood circulation to the muscles. It also opens up the air passages of the body, making it easier to breathe. For this reason, asthmatics, who sometimes suffer attacks when under great stress, are usually given some form of epinephrine to alleviate their symptoms.

The adrenal glands are small, triangular in shape, and can be found draped over the tops of the kidneys. They consist of two main parts. The soft, dark brown inner part is known as the medulla. It produces the hormones epinephrine and norepinephrine. The outer layer, or cortex, is deep yellow in color. It is regulated by the pituitary gland and produces over thirty hormones — classified chemically as steroids — that regulate many of the body's metabolic functions.

Disorders of the adrenal glands fall into two broad categories. Adrenal underproduction, known as hypoadrenalism, is a life-threatening disorder. It cannot be cured but can be controlled with the use of hormonal extracts and artificial hormones. Adrenal overproduction, hyperadrenalism, is often caused by tumors in the adrenal glands or in the related pituitary gland and can exhibit such symptoms as high blood pressure, a continual state of physical alarm, abnormal loss of potassium (which results in muscle weakness and cramping), and heavy salt concentrations in the urine that can cause severe kidney damage. Surgical removal of the tumors will usually bring about a dramatic improvement or even eliminate the symptoms completely.

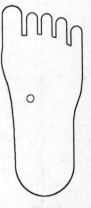

BOTH HANDS

BOTH FEET

The role reflexology plays in the health of the adrenal glands is a preventive one. A workout of the adrenal reflex points on the hands and feet encourages the adrenals in their normal production of hormones and can help maintain their health and resistance to disease. Because there are two adrenal glands, there is a reflex point on the palms of both hands and the soles of both feet. The points on the left hand and foot stimulate the left adrenal gland; the ones on the right hand and foot stimulate the right adrenal gland. The hand reflex point is above the tendon of the thumb, about one-third of the way between the base of the index finger and the wrist. The foot reflex point is near the base of the ball of the foot, below the big toe.

TECHNIQUES

The adrenal areas are fairly small and specific points on both the hands and the feet. Visualize the adrenal gland that you are stimulating and regulate your breathing. Inhale as you press its reflex and exhale as you release the pressure. Work the point slowly and deliberately, but do not cause any real pain. Since there are two adrenal glands, it is best to work on the reflexes for both of them.

THE HANDS — To find the adrenal point on both the right and left palms, place your thumb on the pad beneath your index finger. Gently slide your thumb straight down toward your wrist. Stop just before you reach the inside edge of the pad that extends from the thumb of the hand you are working on. This is the adrenal reflex point. Press firmly on this point, using your thumb. You are going to do this seven times. The first time, press slowly and gently, then let up slightly on the pressure. Be sure not to stop the pressure altogether; just pull back a little. Exert a little more pressure on the second press, then pull back a little again. Increase the pressure each time, but do not stop the pressure completely until you have finished the workout.

THE FEET — To find the adrenal point on the right and left soles, first flex your toes. Notice how a tendon forms a ridge from the ball of your foot to the heel. Move your thumb along this tendon to a point just above the halfway point between the toes and the heel in the arch of the foot. Then, if you are working on your right foot, with the sole of the foot facing you, move your thumb just to the right of the tendon. This is the adrenal reflex point. If you are working on your left foot, the point will be in the corresponding spot just to the left of the tendon. Press firmly on this point with your thumb. Using a technique identical to that for the hand, you are going to do this seven times. Press slowly and gently the first time. Release the pressure slightly but not altogether; just pull back a little. Increase the pressure each time, pulling back between presses. Do not let up on the pressure completely until you have finished the adrenal workout.

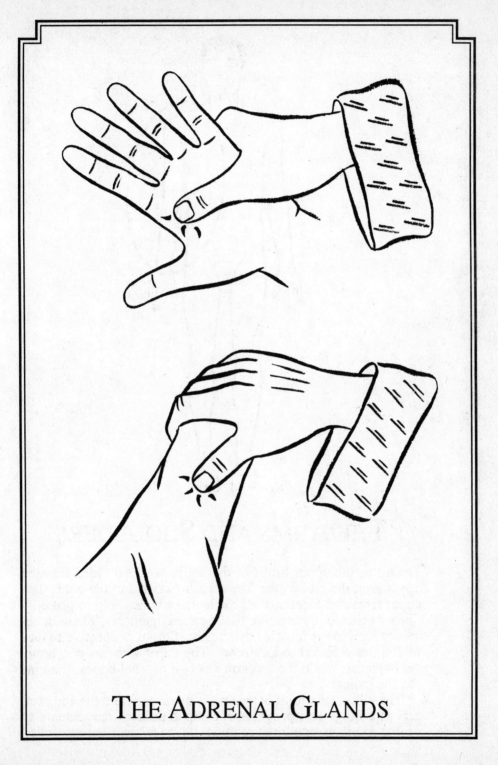

THE ADRENAL GLANDS

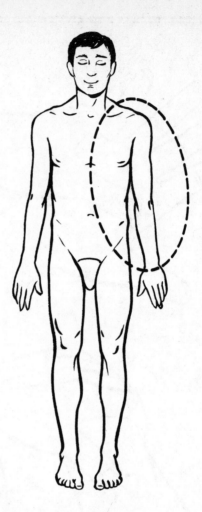

THE ARMS AND SHOULDERS

The arms, the upper limbs of the body, can be divided into the upper arm, the elbow, the forearm, the wrist, and the hand. The upper arms and forearms are made up of bones held in place by fibrous bands of connective tissue called ligaments. These bones are attached to the muscles by tendons, fibrous connective tissues sometimes referred to as sinews. The upper arm has one bone, the humerus, while the forearm has two parallel bones, the ulna and the radius.

The elbow, the joint between the upper arm and the forearm, acts as a hinge and provides both up and down movements as well as a certain amount of rotation. Its movements are controlled by two muscles in the upper arm called the bicep and the tricep. A particularly sensitive nerve, mistakenly named the "funny bone," runs near the surface of the elbow: When struck suddenly, the nerve triggers a tingling sensation in the elbow and other parts of the arm. A small sac of connective tissue called the bursa helps lubricate the joint and make the movement of the elbow smooth and easy. The wrist, at the bottom of the forearm, is made up of eight bones in two rows, cleverly arranged to provide almost complete rotation of the hands.

While the elbow and the wrist are the joints of the arm, the shoulder contains a ball-and-socket joint that connects the arm to the trunk of the body. This joint, located in a shallow cavity on the shoulder blade, is held together by a network of muscles, ligaments, and tendons. Like the hip, the shoulder has a wide range of movement in almost every direction, but it is not as stable as the hip. In fact, the shoulder is the joint most likely to be dislocated in the body.

Because of their location and frequent movement in use, the shoulder and arm are subject to problems ranging from cuts and bruises to broken bones, torn ligaments, sprains, and dislocations. When the bursa in the shoulder or elbow becomes inflamed due to irritation or injury, a painful condition known as bursitis results. This can be treated with cortisone to reduce the swelling, although immobilization of the affected joint, rest, and heat are the most common remedies. Tendonitis, an inflammation of the tendon, is caused by repeated pressure on the tendons in the wrist and forearm from any activity that involves moving a joint while exerting pressure. "Tennis elbow" is one of the more commonly known forms of tendonitis and is treated by putting the arm into a sling to immobilize the elbow.

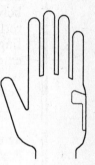

BOTH HANDS

Since the arms are the conduits for the reflexology points on the hands, it should be immediately apparent how important the health of the arms and shoulders can be to the general health of the body. Regular physical exercise is an excellent way to keep the arms and shoulders healthy, and a reflexology workout can help keep them fine-tuned, while alleviating many of the painful conditions that can plague them.

The reflex areas for the arms and shoulders are on both feet and both hands. On each foot, the area starts on the sole, at the crease between the fourth toe and the little toe, goes down to the lower edge of the large pad at the base of the little toe, and extends around onto the outer edge of the foot. On each palm, the area starts at the crease between the ring finger and the little finger, extends down to the lower edge of the pad under that finger, then wraps around onto the outer edge of the hand.

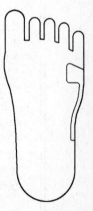

BOTH FEET

TECHNIQUES

The reflex areas on the right hand and foot correspond to the right arm and shoulder, while those on the left hand and foot correspond to the left arm and shoulder. Be sure to work both sides, rather than just one, and be alert for any pain or tenderness in the areas — these may be clues to some form of distress in the arms or shoulders. Work the area slowly, using deliberate pressure but without causing any real pain. Visualize the part of the body that you are working on and inhale as you press the reflex area, exhaling as you release the pressure.

THE HANDS — The arm and shoulder reflex areas on the hands are easy to find. Place your thumb at the base of the crease between the ring finger and the little finger. This is the top of the reflex area. It extends down to just below the pad of the little finger and ranges across onto the edge of the hand. The area then extends down along the edge of the hand, about two-thirds of the way. Use your thumb to work the area on the palm, then, for better leverage, grasp the hand firmly and switch to using your index and middle fingers for the edge. Start with a gentle but firm rolling pressure. Release the pressure just a little, then press again a little harder. You are going to work out the entire reflex area seven times. Do not release the pressure altogether until you have finished the workout.

THE FEET — The arm and shoulder reflex areas on the feet start beneath the crease between the fourth toe and the little toe and extend down to just below the large pad (part of the "ball" of the foot) that is at the base of the little toe. The reflex area ranges across to the outer edge of the foot. It then continues down the edge of the foot to just above the heel pad. Using a technique identical to that for the hands, you are going to work the entire reflex area seven times, using your thumb on the sole and switching to your index and middle fingers for better leverage on the edge of the foot. Press with a gentle but firm, rolling motion the first time. Let up on the pressure just a little, then press again, this time a little harder. Increase the pressure each time, releasing it only slightly between presses. Do not release the pressure completely until the arm and shoulder workout is finished.

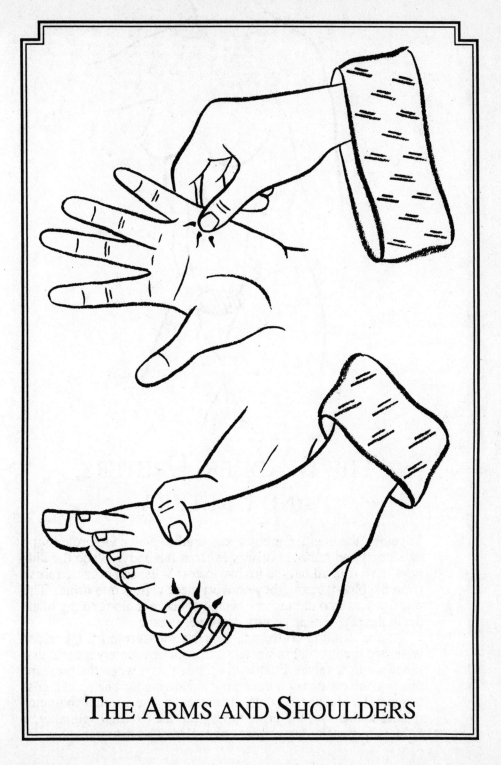

THE ARMS AND SHOULDERS

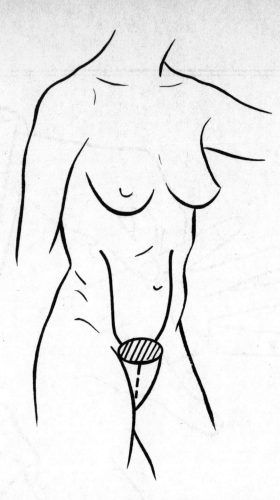

THE BLADDER, URETERS, AND URETHRA

Together, the bladder, ureters, and urethra play a vital role in the collection and removal of wastes from the body. Once the kidneys have filtered out the toxins, excess salts, and organic refuse from the bloodstream, they convert these wastes into urine. The urine passes into the ureters, which squeeze it along to the bladder at the rate of nearly thirty drops per minute.

As the urine is collected, it exerts pressure on the bladder walls and the internal sphincter, a smooth involuntary muscle that functions as a valve. Four to six times a day, when the pressure reaches one-quarter of a pound per square inch, a chemical signal triggers the bladder to empty its contents. The internal sphincter relaxes and passes the urine through to the external sphincter, a voluntary muscle that can be controlled. The external sphincter tightens up and holds back the urine until it is convenient for the person to urinate. Then the sphincter relaxes and the urine flows down a tube known as the urethra and out of the body. While urine gets its yellowish color from bile excreted by the liver, it is actually sterile and odorless until it passes through the urethra. Then the urine is exposed to microorganisms in the environment that break it down into compounds such as ammonia, giving urine its characteristic odor.

The ureters are a pair of muscular tubes the size of a pencil in diameter and ten to twelve inches long. They extend from the kidneys down to the bladder, a balloonlike sac that expands to hold about a pint of urine. The bladder empties into the urethra, which is only about one and a half inches long in women. In men, the urethra is usually eight or nine inches long and passes semen as well as urine out of the body.

There are many types of urinary problems that can develop. Cystitis, very common in women, is an inflammation of the bladder caused by environmental or sexually transmitted organisms that have traveled up the short urethra. Bladder stones are either passed into the bladder from the kidneys or formed in the bladder when the urine becomes too concentrated. They range in size from a microscopic crystal to a hen's egg and hospitalize one out of every thousand people in the United States every year. Incontinence, the inability to control the flow of urine, can be caused by pelvic and sphincter muscles weakened in pregnancy and childbirth or by inadequate development of the bladder sphincters. It also may come during the normal process of aging. NSU, nonspecific urethritis, is an inflammation of the urethra and is especially common in men. Its causes are not really understood, although chlamydia and other such organisms are frequently indicted.

BOTH HANDS

At this time, there is no permanent remedy for bladder stones, but a workout of the bladder reflexes can help keep it active enough to regularly flush itself out, passing smaller stones and preventing a buildup of overconcentrated urine. This can also exercise the sphincters to prevent or cut down on incidences of incontinence. By increasing the blood circulation to the ureters, bladder, and urethra, muscular development is encouraged and resistance to infections is increased.

The reflex areas for the ureters, bladder, and urethra are on the palms of both hands and the soles of both feet. The hand reflex area ranges from the inner edge of the large pad below the thumb down to the outer, lower edge of the palm. On the foot the area ranges from the middle of the soft hollow in the arch to the inner edge of the foot, next to the pad of the heel.

BOTH FEET

TECHNIQUES

There is a strong interrelationship among the ureters, bladder, and urethra, and it is best to stimulate the reflex area for all three in the same session. You will find reflex areas on the palms of both hands and the soles of both feet, as there are ureters on both sides of the body. Also, because the bladder and urethra are in the center of the body, their reflex areas are actually split between the two hands and the two feet. Always work both sides of the body for best results.

THE HANDS — The reflex area for the ureter, bladder, and urethra on both the right and left palms is not difficult to find. Place your thumb at the crease between the index and middle fingers and move it straight down toward the wrist until you are on the inside edge of the large pad at the base of the thumb. This is the beginning of the ureter reflex. Look at the area of your palm where the pad joins the wrist. Just to the left of this on the left palm (just to the right on the right palm) is a slight bump on the edge of the hand. This is the bladder/urethra reflex. Perform a firm, rolling squeeze on the area, working from the inner ureter point down to the bladder/urethra reflex. You are going to do this seven times. Squeeze and roll slowly and gently with your thumb the first time, then release the pressure slightly. Increase your thumb pressure with each subsequent rolling squeeze, but do not let up on the pressure completely until you have finished.

THE FEET — On the foot the reflex point for the ureter is in the middle of the soft hollow in the arch, straight down from the second toe. The bladder/urethra reflex is at the lower end of the arch on the edge of the foot, next to the pad of the heel. You are going to massage the area extending from the beginning of the ureter reflex over to the bladder/urethra reflex seven times, using an identical technique to that for the hand. Start at the ureter reflex and use your thumb to exert a firm, rolling squeeze down to the bladder/urethra reflex area. Do this gently the first time, then let up on the pressure slightly. Increase the pressure with each rolling squeeze. Pull back between squeezes, but do not stop exerting pressure until the bladder workout is completed.

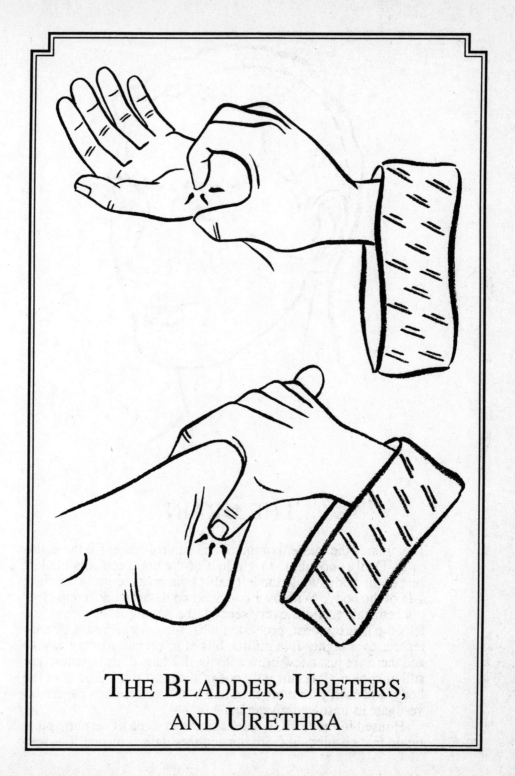

THE BLADDER, URETERS, AND URETHRA

The Brain

The brain is the master computer and control center for the entire body. Oddly enough, the right half of the brain controls the left side of the body, while the left half of the brain controls the right side of the body. With over one hundred thousand different electrochemical reactions every second, the brain houses memories, tells the heart to beat, processes what the eyes and ears take in, records over eighty-five million bits of information every day — and these are just a few of its activities! Many of its functions are still unknown. It is currently one of the most studied parts of the body, and each year more than half a million research papers investigate its unsolved mysteries.

Housed in the skull, where it floats in a sea of cerebrospinal liquid that cushions it from impact, the brain is made up of several parts. Some of these are: the spinal bulb (medulla oblongata), which controls vital automatic body functions such as heartbeat and breathing; the cerebellum, which controls balance and co-ordinates muscle actions; and the hypothalamus, which determines the water balance in the body, body temperature, and sleep patterns, as well as basic drives such as hunger, pleasure, anger, and sexual interest.

The largest part of the brain, the one people visualize when the word *brain* is mentioned, is the cerebrum. The cerebrum controls such varied operations as speech, sensation, awareness, personality, and intellect. It consists of two hemispheres, commonly referred to as the left and right brains. While both hemispheres share many common functions, research over the past thirty years has turned up evidence of specialization in each one. The left hemisphere processes information linearly and dominates verbal and analytical skills such as reading, writing, speech, and logic. The right hemisphere processes information in a holistic fashion, grasping the relationships between things rather than individual items. It is nonverbal but dominates spatial relations, visual imagery, and pattern recognition. While the right brain cannot produce speech, it can understand it. Images in dreams or in the "mind's eye" come from the right brain, as well as perceptions of depth, music, color, and facial recognition.

There are many problems that can affect some or all of the brain's neurologic functions. Some are degenerative diseases, such as Alzheimer's, in which memory patterns are lost, and Parkinson's, in which muscle control degenerates. Others are traumatic, such as concussion — a temporary loss of consciousness or a dazed feeling due to the violent shaking the brain receives from a blow to the head; or laceration — actual damage done to the brain, which can result in permanent impairment. One serious neurologic disability is apoplexy, or stroke — a sudden interruption of the blood circulation in the brain. The two most common types of stroke are embolism, the blockage of an artery by a bloodclot, air bubble, or fat particle; and hemorrhage, the rupture of a blood vessel in the brain, often caused by high blood pressure.

A workout of the brain's reflex areas can help keep it active and alert. The brain reflex area on the hands is the tip of each thumb. On the feet it is the tip of each big toe. There is one additional detail — since the right side of the brain controls the left side of the body and the left side of the brain controls the right side of the body, stimulating the right toe or thumb affects the left side of the body, and stimulating the left toe or thumb affects the right side of the body.

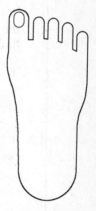

BOTH HANDS

BOTH FEET

TECHNIQUES

To stimulate the left side of the brain, work the reflexes of the right hand or foot; to stimulate the right side of the brain, work the reflexes on the left hand or foot. The right hemisphere of the brain controls such intellectual functions as spatial orientation and creativity, while the left controls analytical abilities and speech. It is important, when working on the brain reflexes, to remember that the brain has a crossover effect on the body—the right half of the brain affects the functions of the left side of the body, and the left half of the brain affects the functions of the right side of the body. Visualize the part of the brain that you are working on and regulate your breathing. Inhale as you press the reflex and exhale as you release the pressure. Note any tenderness—this may be a clue to some form of distress. Be careful not to cause any real discomfort as you work the area.

THE HANDS — The brain reflex area on both hands is the tip of the thumb and the area just below the tip. Grasp the tip of the thumb between your thumb and index finger. Perform a firm, rolling squeeze or pinch on the area, slowly moving all the way around the tip. You are going to do this seven times. First, squeeze and roll gently but firmly, then release the pressure slightly. Do not let up on the pressure completely; just ease it a little. Increase the pressure with each rolling squeeze, releasing it only slightly until you have finished the workout.

THE FEET — On both feet the brain reflex area is the tip of the big toe and the area just below the tip. Grasp it between your thumb and index finger and perform a firm, rolling squeeze as you move around to cover the entire reflex area. You are going to do this seven times in a technique identical to the one for the hand. Squeeze and roll gently but firmly at first, then release the pressure slightly. Press a little harder on the second rolling squeeze, then pull back again. Continue to increase the pressure with each subsequent rolling squeeze, but do not release the pressure completely until the brain workout is completed.

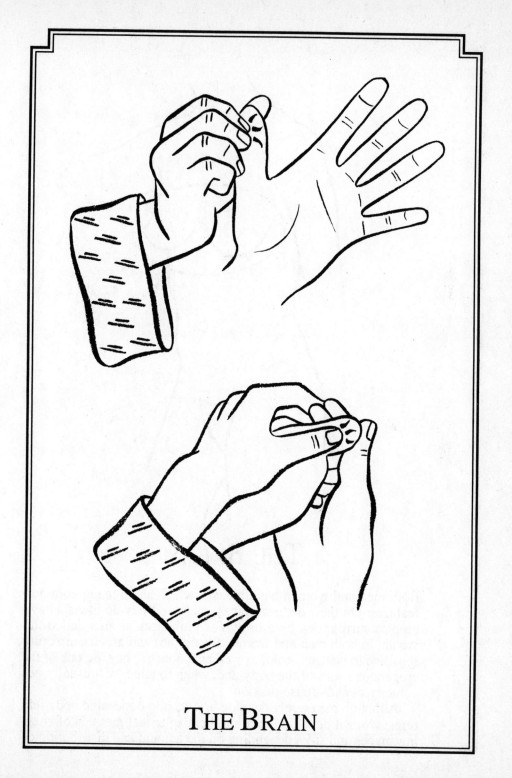

THE BRAIN

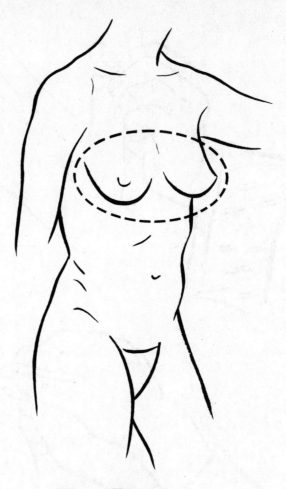

THE BREASTS

Both men and women have breasts, which share many common features. On their outer surfaces, male and female breasts have nipples surrounded by a brown or pink circular area called the areola. In both men and women the nipples and areolae are quite sensitive to heat and cold, as well as to touch. They are one of the erogenous zones of the body and, when fondled, will usually become erect and arouse passion.

Although men rarely develop breasts into noticeable body features, women develop them into hemispherical mounds of varying shapes and sizes depending on the amount and distribution of the fat cells from which they are composed. It is not unusual for a woman to have breasts that are not matched in size or shape. In fact, women will often find that their left breast is slightly larger than their right breast. Although breasts are designed to feed babies, breast size does not determine either sexual responsiveness or the amount of milk a breast can produce.

Besides fat, the inside of the breast contains connective tissue and a mammary gland made up of ducts and nodes that are milk-producing areas. The breast begins to develop at puberty, when a great increase in sex hormones triggers the growth of glandular tissue. As a female matures, fat starts to collect around the ducts and milk-producing areas, increasing the size of the breast. How much fat accumulates is determined by many factors: Heredity, hormonal balances, and changes in body weight are just a few. Breasts usually reach their largest size during pregnancy and breast-feeding periods, when the milk-producing areas are at their peak and the glandular ducts are full. In later life, as a woman reaches menopause and its accompanying hormonal changes, the breasts shrink in size and change in texture.

The most dangerous disease of the breast is cancer. According to the American Cancer Society, one woman out of eleven in the United States will develop some form of breast cancer, and of these, one woman out of three will die of it, a mortality statistic that has not changed significantly since 1930. Causes of breast cancer are still a mystery, although both heredity and a high-fat diet are suspected. Successful survival of the disease seems to be dependent on early detection (by means such as regular self-examination of the breasts) and treatment (usually a combination of surgery and chemotherapy).

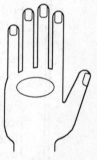

BOTH HANDS

One of the most common problems with the breast is swelling and tenderness for a few days prior to a menstrual period. This is due to hormonal changes that cause the temporary retention of water. Inflammation of the mammary gland, known as mastitis, occurs in nursing mothers and is usually due to infection. A fibrocystic condition, often mistakenly called fibrocystic "disease," exists when the breasts have tender lumps formed by sacs of gelatinous or fluid matter under the surface of the breasts. These cysts are usually benign, are not uncommon, and seem to be hormonally dependent.

A workout of the breast reflex areas on the hands and feet can help maintain their health and resistance to disease. The breast reflex areas on each hand are not on the palm but on the back of the hand, starting just below the knuckles and extending down for a few inches. On the top of each foot, the reflex area starts just above the toes and extends toward the ankle a few inches.

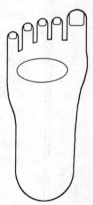

BOTH FEET

TECHNIQUES

The breast reflex areas are located on the back of each hand and the top of each foot. Work these areas carefully, as they are extremely sensitive to pressure and can be easily bruised. Take your time and work the area thoroughly, paying particular attention to any sore spots, which may indicate that some sort of distress is present. Visualize the part of the body that you are working on and regulate your breathing. Inhale as you press the reflex, and exhale as you release the pressure.

THE HANDS — The breast reflex area is on the back of both hands, from the knuckles at the bases of the fingers to about halfway to the wrist. The area ranges across the hand from below the little finger to just below the index finger. Put your thumb in the center of your palm for resistance. Wrap your fingers around your hand and, moving your index, middle, and ring fingers in a circular, rolling motion, press gently as you move along the area. Be sure to work the entire area, including the spots between the bones and tendons. You are going to do the entire area seven times, increasing the pressure each time. Remember that the right hand corresponds to the right breast and the left hand to the left breast; but it is always a good idea to work both hands.

THE FEET — The breast reflex area is on the top of each of foot. It extends from the base of the toes to about halfway to the ankle, and ranges from the second toe across the top of the foot. You are going to stimulate the entire area seven times, using a technique similar to that for the hands. Put the palm of your hand against the sole for resistance, and use your index and middle fingers in a circular, rolling motion. Press gently as you move along the area, carefully including the spots between the bones and tendons. Increase the pressure each time, but do not press too hard. Although the area on the right foot stimulates the right breast and the area on the left foot stimulates the left breast, it is a good idea to work on both sides.

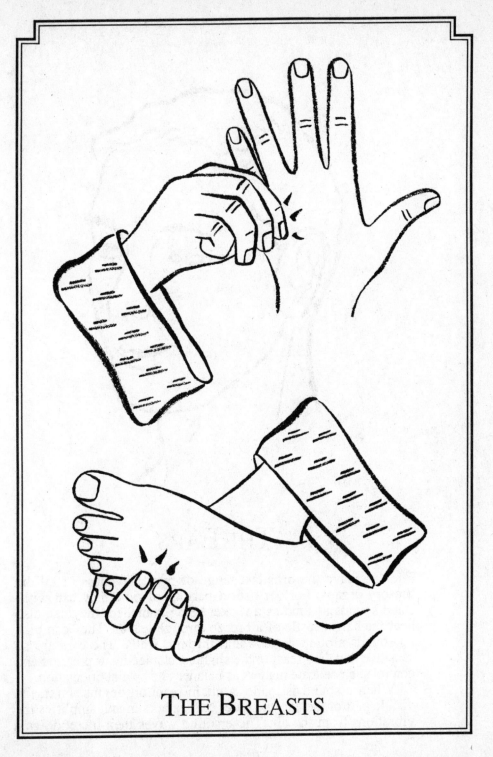

THE BREASTS

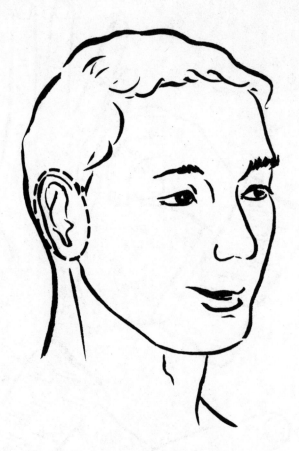

THE EARS

The ears have the broadest range of responsiveness of all the sensory organs. For very short periods of time they can withstand sounds as loud as a rocket being launched; they can also hear the barest rustle of a breeze through leaves. They can pick up sounds around corners and through walls. The ears are so sensitive that they react to the slightest change in air pressure and control such delicate matters as balance and spatial orientation.

When a sound is made, a chain reaction begins. First, the visible part of the ear, the outer ear, gathers in and amplifies the vibrations from the air. These sound waves then travel down a short tunnel to reach a half-inch-wide, paper-thin membrane known as the tympanic membrane, or eardrum. Attached to the inner surface of the eardrum is the air-filled middle ear containing three tiny bones, called, because of their shapes, the hammer, anvil, and stirrup. The middle ear is connected to the back of the throat by the eustachian tube, which causes the pressure inside the middle ear to be the same as the pressure on the outside. When the sound waves reach the eardrum, it flutters up to two-billionths of an inch, causing the tiny ear bones to move in response and send their message along to the inner ear, a snail-shell-shaped structure of fluid-filled chambers called the cochlea. The fluid in the chambers reacts to the pulsing of the middle ear bones and triggers the auditory nerve to send a signal to the au-ditory center of the brain, where it is analyzed and identified.

The inner ear also contains three semicircular canals that control the sense of equilibrium. These fluid-filled canals are set at right angles to each other and function like spinning wheels in a gyroscope. The fluid is at rest when the body is upright. When the body moves quickly or leans, the fluid moves accordingly and sends a message to the brain, which then notifies the muscles to maintain balance. Motion sickness may occur when the fluids in the semicircular canals are in a sustained state of turbulence.

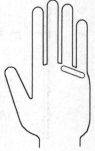

One common ear problem is tinnitus, a ringing or hissing in the ear caused by factors ranging from damage to the inner ear to psychological disorders. Another is swimmer's ear, an infection from microorganisms in water that has entered the ear. By far the most common problem is an earache that results from upper-respiratory infections, usually caused by germs from infected mucus that have entered the eustachian tube from the back of the throat. Earaches can also be caused by blowing the nose too hard. At least half the children under five years of age have suffered an earache from this form of infection. Other ear prob-lems are triggered by trauma, such as a sudden change in air pressure, a slap across the ear, or an explosively loud sound — all of which can rupture the eardrum. These, along with loud sounds over a sustained period of time, as well as the process of aging, can result in temporary or permanent deafness.

BOTH HANDS

A reflexology workout of the ears can help maintain their health and, in some cases, can alleviate motion sickness. Since there are two ears, the ear reflex points are on the palms of both hands and the soles of both feet. The points on the right hand and foot correspond to the right ear, while those on the left hand and foot correspond to the left ear. The hand reflex point is at the base of the ring finger and the little finger. On the foot, the point is at the base of the fourth toe and the little toe.

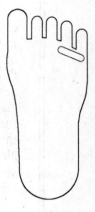

BOTH FEET

TECHNIQUES

The ear reflex on both the hands and the feet is a small area rather than a specific point. Be sure to note any tenderness when exerting pressure on this area. This tenderness may be a clue to some form of distress, so work the point slowly and deliberately, but be careful not to cause any real pain. Visualize the ear as you work on its reflex, and regulate your breathing. Inhale as you press, and exhale as you release the pressure. Since there are two ears, there are points on both the right and left hands and feet that correspond to the right and left ears. It is best to work on both ears rather than concentrating on only one of them in a workout session.

THE HANDS — The ear reflex on both the right and left palms is at the base of the ring finger and little finger, and includes the webbing between them. Place your thumb firmly on the palm of your hand in this area, with your index finger opposing it, as though you were going to pinch the webbing between the fingers. Perform a firm, rolling squeeze on the area, a movement not unlike trying to rub some paint off your palm. You are going to do this seven times. The first time, squeeze and roll slowly and gently, then release the pressure slightly. Do not stop the pressure altogether; just pull back a little. On subsequent squeezes, increase the pressure each time, pulling back between squeezes. Do not let up on the pressure completely until you have finished.

THE FEET — The ear reflexes on the right and left feet are on the soles, at the base of the fourth toe and the little toe, and include the webbing between them. Place your thumb on the sole of your foot at this point and, as though you were going to pinch the webbing between the toes, put your index finger opposite your thumb. Exert a firm, rolling squeeze on the area. You are going to do this seven times, using a technique identical to that for the hand. The first time, squeeze and roll slowly and gently, then release the pressure slightly, but do not stop the pressure altogether. For the subsequent squeezes, gently increase the pressure each time, pulling back between squeezes. Do not let up on the pressure completely until you have finished the ear workout.

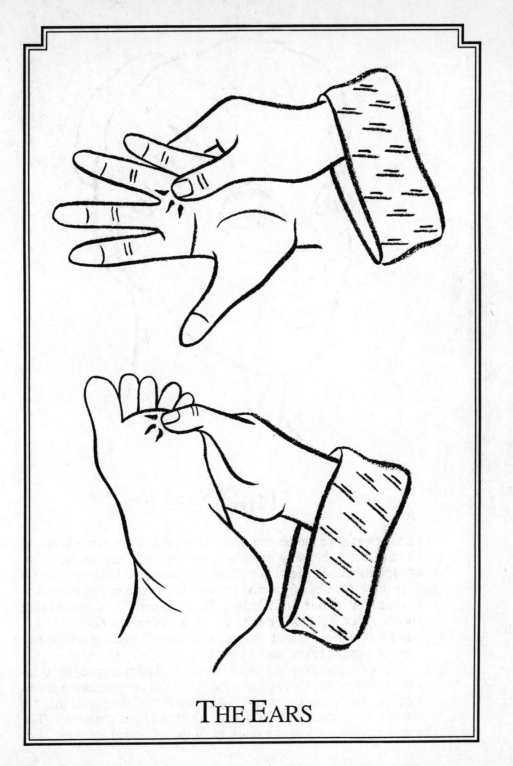

THE EARS

THE EYES

The eyes expose the central nervous system to the external world more directly than any other sensory organ. They are sensitive enough to take in over ten million gradations of light and absorb over three-fourths of the raw sensory information that forms the foundation of our knowledge. This happens at a remarkable speed: After light first enters the eyes, there is a delay of only one-five-hundredth of a second (the time it takes a balloon to pop) before the brain "sees" an object.

The eye functions just like a one-inch-diameter spherical camera. Light passes through an outer lens, the cornea, into a round opening known as the pupil. The diameter of the pupil, like the shutter of a camera, varies according to the light's intensity. The pupil is controlled by the muscles of the iris surrounding it. Behind the pupil and iris is another lens, which focuses the light on the back of the eye, or retina. The retina, which acts like the film in a camera, is a network of fine nerve cells known as rods and cones. They are very tiny — there are one hundred million rods and ten million cones in the retina of each eye. They make it possible for the eye to develop two pictures at once — rods take a black-and-white picture, cones a color picture. Each one of the rods and cones is attached to a long nerve fiber. When light reaches the retina, the rods and cones send their messages through the nerve fibers, or axons, to a point directly behind the retina. There the axons join together to form the optic nerve. There are no cones and rods at the place where the optic nerve joins the retina, hence its name — the blind spot. The optic nerve receives the signal and sends it on to the brain, which translates the signal into visual information.

A perfectly formed eye is shaped like a sphere, and the cornea and lens will focus light directly to a specific point on the retina. If the eyeball's axis is too long or the refractive (bending) power of the lens is too strong, the focal point for the lens will fall in front of the retina and the eye will be nearsighted. If the axis is too short or the refractive power of the lens is too weak, the focal point of the lens falls behind the retina and the eye will be farsighted. In cases of astigmatism, where the cornea and lens have differences in curvature, parallel rays of light are focused at different angles on the retina, making vision blurry. All these conditions are usually corrected by wearing glasses or contact lenses, and, in many cases, new surgical techniques such as radial keratotomy and lens and corneal transplants are available for permanent correction.

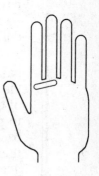

BOTH HANDS

The most common eye problems are: cataracts, the clouding of the lens, which is especially common in the elderly; glaucoma, a condition in which there is too much pressure within the eye; infections, due to microorganisms; detached retina, where the retina has become separated from the underlying layers of the eye; and atrophy of the optic nerve. Most of these conditions can be treated if discovered quickly.

A reflexology workout can stimulate the eyes to stay healthy and resist infections and may help alleviate many eye problems. Since there are two eyes, the eye reflex points can be found on the palms of both hands and soles of both feet. The points on the left hand and foot correspond to the left eye, and the points on the right hand and foot correspond to the right eye. The foot reflex is the area on the sole at the base of the second and third toes. On the hand, the reflex is the area on the palm at the base of the index and middle fingers.

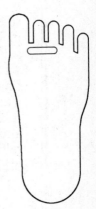

BOTH FEET

TECHNIQUES

Because there are two eyes, there are reflexes on both the right and left hands and feet. The reflex areas on the left hand and foot stimulate the left eye, while the ones on the right hand and foot stimulate the right eye. It is best to work on both eyes rather than concentrating on only one of them in a session. The eye reflex on both the hands and the feet is a small area rather than a specific point. Breathe in as you press the reflex, breathe out as you release the pressure, and visualize the eye and its visual processes while you are working on its reflex. Note carefully any tenderness when exerting pressure on the reflex, as this tenderness may be a clue to some form of distress. Work the area slowly and deliberately, but be careful not to cause any real pain.

THE HANDS — The eye reflex on both the right and left palms is at the base of the index and middle fingers, and includes the webbing between them. Place your thumb firmly on this part of the palm of your hand, using your fingers on the opposite side to provide resistance. Perform a firm, rolling squeeze, moving back and forth to cover the entire reflex area. You are going to do this seven times. The first time, squeeze and roll slowly and gently with your thumb, then release the pressure slightly. Increase the pressure with each squeeze, and do not let up on the pressure completely until you have finished the eye workout.

THE FEET — The eye reflex areas on the right and left soles of the feet are at the base of the second and third toes, and include the webbing between them. Place your fingertips on the sole of your foot in this area and use your thumb on the opposite side to provide resistance. Exert a firm, rolling squeeze with your fingers, moving back and forth over the entire eye reflex area. You are going to do this seven times. The first time, squeeze and roll gently, then release the pressure slightly, but do not stop it altogether. Increase the pressure with each squeeze and roll, releasing it slightly between squeezes, but do not stop exerting pressure until the eye workout is finished.

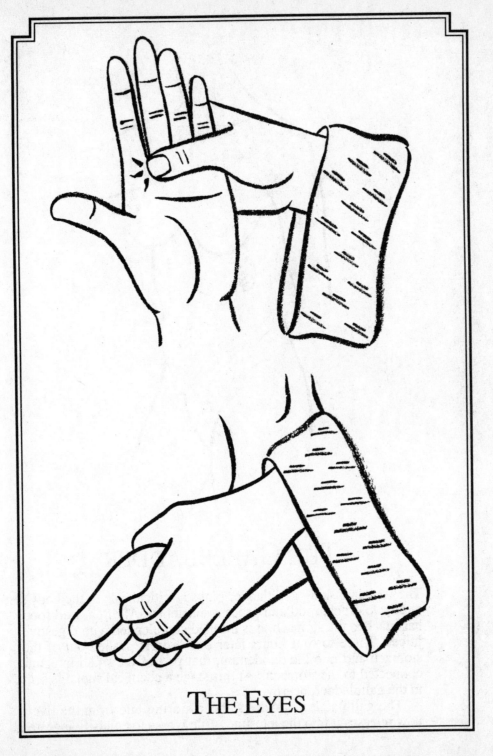

THE EYES

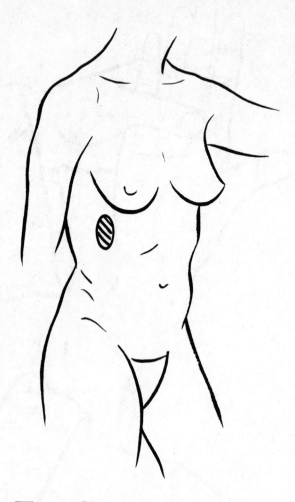

THE GALLBLADDER

The four-inch-long gallbladder plays a critical role in the body's ability to digest food and process nutrients. After chewed food has reached the stomach, it is mashed and blended with digestive juices. Three to four hours later this food is pushed out of the stomach and into the duodenum, that part of the small intestine connected to the stomach. At this stage a chemical signal is sent to the gallbladder, nearby.

The gallbladder, which has been storing bile from the liver, now releases it into the intestine. Bile works to emulsify ingested fats, allowing them to be absorbed into the body, and is essential for the absorption of important fat-soluble vitamins. Among these are vitamin A, which is necessary for good night vision, healthy skin and hair, and the prevention of tooth decay; vitamin D, which promotes healthy bones and teeth; vitamin E, which prevents the oxidation of unsaturated fats, thus preserving and rejuvenating tissue; and vitamin K, a key component in normal blood clotting. Furthermore, bile acts as a deodorizer and a mild laxative by encouraging the intestine to move the food along instead of allowing it to sit and ferment.

The gallbladder is a pear-shaped receptacle nestled behind the right side of the liver. The liver manufactures the yellow-brown bile, and it is the gallbladder that stores and concentrates it until it is needed. Sometimes the concentration of bile can cause problems for the gallbladder. If the bile becomes too concentrated, small particles may precipitate out to form gallstones. One out of every ten people suffers from gallstones and one-fifth of the population over forty years of age is plagued by them. Sometimes gallstones seem to cause no problem; at other times their presence is announced by excruciating pain.

There are two basic kinds of gallstones — those that are calcium-based and those that are composed of crystallized cholesterol. No one understands quite how or why they are formed, but surgery is the most common treatment, especially for gallstones that are calcium-based. Cholesterol-based stones respond to some of the newer drug treatments. A fifteen-year research study at the Mayo Clinic determined that taking bile orally over a period of time dissolved cholesterol-based gallstones. It may be that ingested bile stimulates the liver either to secrete more bile acids or to cut down on its cholesterol secretion.

A workout of the gallbladder reflex can help to keep it alert and active. An active gallbladder will flush itself out and is less likely to have a buildup of sludge from overconcentrated bile. In cases where gallstones are present, stimulating the gallbladder reflex points may cut down on the incidence of painful stone attacks by causing the gall duct to relax enough to pass the stones into the small intestine and out of the body altogether.

Because the gallbladder is located on the right side of the body, the reflex points are found only on the right hand and the right foot. On the hand, the point is on the palm, located down from the crease between the ring finger and the little finger, about one-third of the way between the base of the fingers and the wrist. On the foot, this point can be found on the sole, almost directly under the crease between the fourth toe and the little toe, about halfway to the heel.

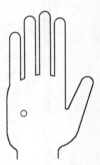

RIGHT HAND

RIGHT FOOT

TECHNIQUES

The gallbladder reflex on both the hand and the foot is a fairly small and specific point. When exerting pressure on the reflex, be sure to note any tenderness. Work the point slowly and deliberately, but be careful not to cause any real pain. Visualize the gallbladder as you are working on its reflex, and imagine it functioning efficiently. Coordinate your breathing with the workout by inhaling as you press the reflex and exhaling as you release the pressure.

THE HAND — To find the gallbladder point, gently slide your thumb down the palm of your right hand from the crease between your ring finger and little finger. Stop when you have covered about one-third of the distance between your fingers and your wrist. This is the gallbladder reflex point. Using your thumb, press firmly on this point. You are going to do this seven times. The first time, press slowly and gently, then release the pressure slightly. Do not stop the pressure altogether; just pull back a little. On subsequent presses, increase the pressure each time, pulling back only slightly between presses but never really stopping the pressure until you have finished the workout.

THE FOOT — To find the gallbladder point, gently slide your thumb down the sole of your right foot. Start at the crease between your fourth toe and your little toe. Stop when you have covered a little less than half the distance between your toes and the back of your heel. This is the gallbladder reflex point. Using your thumb, press firmly on this point. You are going to do this seven times, using a technique identical to that for the hand. The first time, press slowly and gently, then release the pressure slightly. Do not stop the pressure altogether, just pull back a little. On the second press, exert a little more pressure on the foot. Pull back a little again. On subsequent presses, increase the pressure each time, pulling back between presses. Do not let up on the pressure completely until you have finished the workout.

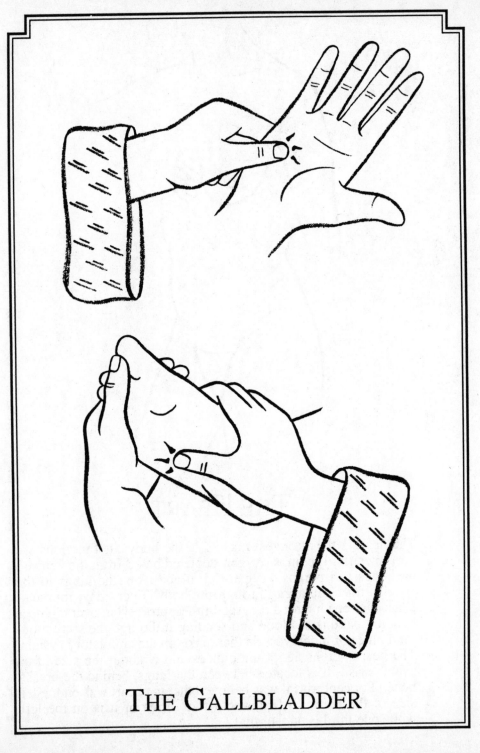

THE GALLBLADDER

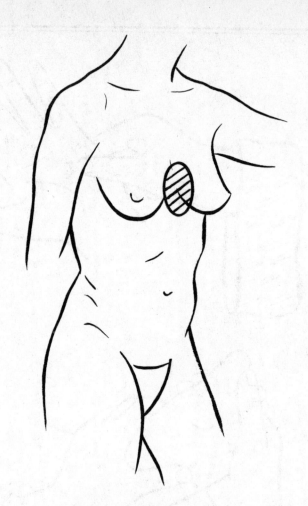

THE HEART

The heart is the strongest muscle in the body. Its functions are very specific: It pumps oxygen-depleted blood from the veins to the lungs and pumps oxygen-rich blood from the lungs to the arteries for circulation through the body. Every day, the heart beats over one hundred thousand times, processing over eighteen hundred gallons of blood and sending it through the sixty thousand miles of blood vessels that make up the circulatory system. The heart weighs about ten ounces and is about the size of an average fist. It is located between the lungs, behind the breastbone. For centuries it was believed that the heart was on the left side of the body. In fact, about two-thirds of it is on the left, while one-third is on the right.

The heart is made up of four distinct chambers separated by four valves. Blood that has circulated through the body and has had its oxygen and other nutrients removed (so-called blue blood) returns to the heart through the veins. It is received by the first chamber, the right atrium. From there the blood is pumped to the second chamber, the right ventricle, which sends it on to the lungs to be oxygenated. On its return trip from the lungs the now bright-red blood is taken in by the left atrium and passed below to the left ventricle, which pumps it out to the arteries and through the body. The heart's pumping cycle, referred to as the cardiac cycle, has two phases — the systolic or pumping phase, and the diastolic or resting phase. When blood pressure is measured, it is usually described as the ratio of systolic pressure to diastolic pressure.

Diseases of the heart are among the major causes of death in the United States. The most common, atherosclerosis, is the narrowing and eventual blockage of an artery by fat deposits, called plaques, on its inner wall. Atherosclerosis develops over time and is primarily related to bad diet and inadequate exercise. When a coronary artery becomes partially blocked by plaques, it often causes chest pain known as angina. If the blockage is complete or if the coronary artery is even temporarily blocked by a blood clot, part of the heart may actually die from lack of oxygen. When this happens, a person is said to suffer a myocardial infarction, or heart attack. When the blocked artery is one leading to the brain, a stroke may occur, damaging or destroying a part of the brain.

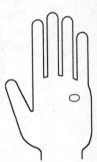

LEFT HAND

There are many other forms of heart problems. Arrhythmia, or irregular heartbeats, is caused by a faulty sinoatrial node, known as the pacemaker, which controls the cardiac cycle's rhythm. Hypertensive heart disease is a disorder caused by high blood pressure, often resulting from prolonged stress, and can manifest itself as a cerebral hemorrhage. Heart murmur occurs when one of the heart valves does not close completely during a cardiac cycle. Congenital heart disease, the general name for over forty types of birth defects of the heart and blood vessels, is present in about ten babies out of every thousand live births. Causes are unknown, although exposure during the early stages of pregnancy to German measles (rubella), radiation, or certain drugs may account for many congenital heart defects.

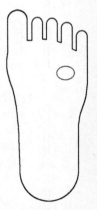

LEFT FOOT

A reflexology workout stimulates the heart to perform its cardiovascular functions and maintain its overall health. The heart reflex points are found on the left palm and the left sole. The reflex point on the palm is just below the pads of the ring finger and little finger. On the sole it is just below the ball of the foot and under the fourth toe.

TECHNIQUES

Since most of the heart is primarily on the left side of the body, its reflexes are found only on the left palm and left sole. While a general massage of the area around the heart reflex is beneficial and desirable, concentration on the reflex itself will yield the most direct results. Whether you are working on the hand or on the foot, the heart reflex will respond equally well. Be sure to note carefully any tenderness in the reflex area, as this may indicate that some form of distress is present. Visualize the heart and its pumping functions as you are stimulating its reflex and imagine your pulse growing stronger and more regular. Regulate your breathing pattern so that you inhale as you press on the reflex and exhale as you release the pressure. Work the area slowly and deliberately, but be careful not to cause any discomfort.

THE HAND — The heart reflex is located on the palm of the left hand. It is just below the pads of the ring finger and little finger. Using your thumb in a circular motion, press gently but firmly on the point. You are going to do this seven times. The first time, exert only a little pressure, then release it slightly. Exert a little more pressure on the second press, then let up a little again. On the subsequent presses, increase your pressure each time, backing off slightly between them. Do not let up on the pressure completely until you have finished the heart workout.

THE FOOT — You will find the heart reflex on the sole of your left foot. Using your right hand to flex the toes, place your left thumb just below the ball of the foot, straight down from the fourth toe. Using a technique identical to that for the hand, use your thumb in a circular motion to press gently and firmly on the reflex seven times. Exert only a little pressure the first time, then release it slightly. On the second press, exert a little more pressure, releasing it slightly again. Increase the pressure on subsequent presses, backing off only slightly between each one. Be sure not to release the pressure completely until you have finished the heart workout.

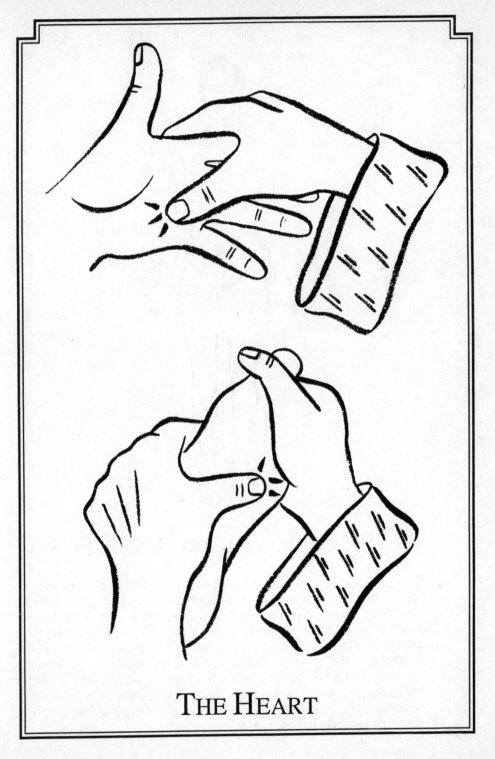

THE HEART

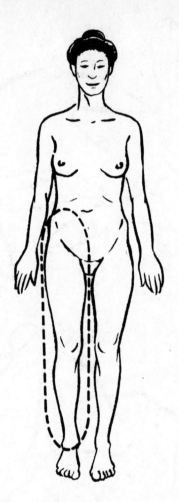

THE HIPS, THIGHS, AND LEGS

The legs, the body's longest limbs, extend from the feet to the hips. The hips connect the legs and buttock area to the trunk of the body. Technically, the leg refers only to that part of the lower limb between the knee and the ankle; the thigh is that part between the hip and the knee. The muscles of the leg and thigh are attached to the bones by tendons — strong, fibrous connective tissues. The thigh has one bone, the femur, which is the longest and strongest bone in the body, while the leg has two, the fibula and the tibia. These bones are held in place by another type of connective tissue called ligaments.

The ankle and the knee are the joints of the leg, while the hip is the joint between the entire lower limb and the body. The ankle is a hinged joint between the foot and the leg that has a range of both up-and-down and side-to-side movements. It glides on a cushion of cartilage — a gelatinous, stretchy type of connective tissue. The knee is the hinge that joins the leg and the thigh. The knee's range of movement makes it one of the most versatile of the hinge joints in the body, surpassing even the fingers or the elbow. It is protected by a cushioning sac known as the bursa, which lies in front of the kneecap, or patella. The hip is a ball-and-socket joint where the upper end of the thighbone fits into the socket of a wing-shaped bone, called the ilium, or hipbone, which is in turn attached to the lower spine. The hip is well padded on the back by muscles that support the weight of the body while sitting. As a joint, the hip is a stronger and more stable ball-and-socket joint than the shoulder, and, while it is sometimes dislocated at birth, it takes a forcible injury to dislocate the hip when it is mature.

The largest nerves of the body, the sciatic nerves, travel down from the hip area through the lower limbs. These nerves play a very important role in the lower limbs, and damage to them can be painful and even result in paralysis. Fractures of the bones in the lower limbs are common occurrences. The hipbones in older people, whose bones have become brittle due to aging, are often broken in falls. In fact, over eighty thousand hips are replaced by artificial substitutes every year in the United States. Knee and ankle bones are often broken in sports and through accidents, such as a false step while walking down stairs. Water on the knee, a painful condition, is an inflammation that causes the kneecap to float. Other problems that affect the lower limbs include bursitis, the inflammation of the bursa due to irritation or injury, especially in the knee and hip; arthritis, a chronic inflammation of the joints; varicose veins, veins that have become swollen and knotted; and torn or detached muscles, sprains, or muscle cramps.

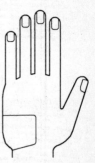

BOTH HANDS

Working the reflexes for the hips and lower limbs can help them heal when they have been hurt and can raise their resistance to infection and injury. Since the lower limbs conduct electro-chemical messages from reflexology points on the feet to the rest of the body, it is readily apparent just how important the health of the lower limbs are to the body in general. The reflex area on each hand is on the lower third of the back of the hand, just above the wrist, down from the ring finger and little finger. On each foot, the area is on the outer edge, about one-third of the way between the heel and the base of the toes.

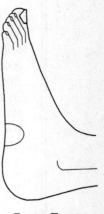

BOTH FEET

TECHNIQUES

Stimulating the reflexes for the hips, thighs, and legs is a great way to invigorate them. The reflexes on the right hand and foot correspond to the right hip, thigh, and leg, while the reflexes on the left hand and foot correspond to the left side. It is a good idea, however, to work on both sides of the body rather than focusing on one. Take your time and work the reflex areas slowly and deliberately. Visualize the part of the body that you are working on and inhale as you press the reflex, then exhale as you release the pressure. Soreness in the reflexes can indicate problems in the hip, thigh, or leg being worked on.

THE HANDS — The hip and lower-limb reflex areas are on the backs of both hands. The area extends from the wrist, up about one-third of the way to the bases of the fingers, and ranges from below the crease between the middle and ring fingers over to the edge of the hand. Use your index, middle, and ring fingers in a circular motion to apply a firm pressure on the area. You are going to cover the entire reflex area seven times in the workout. At first, apply a gentle pressure, then release it slightly. On the next press, increase your pressure, again releasing it slightly. Keep increasing your pressure as you go, releasing a little in between presses. Do not let up completely on the pressure until you have finished the workout.

THE FEET — The reflex area for the hip, thigh, and leg can be found on the outer edge of each foot, about one-third of the way between the heel and the base of the toes, extending from the sole, up to about half the distance to the base of the ankle bone. You are going to use a technique identical to that for the hands, as you stimulate the reflex area on each foot seven times. Use your index and middle fingers in a firm, circular pressing motion to work the edges of the feet. Be sure to work the areas of both feet for the best results. Start with a gentle pressure. Increase the pressure every time you press, but do not release the pressure entirely until the hip, thigh, and leg workout is completed.

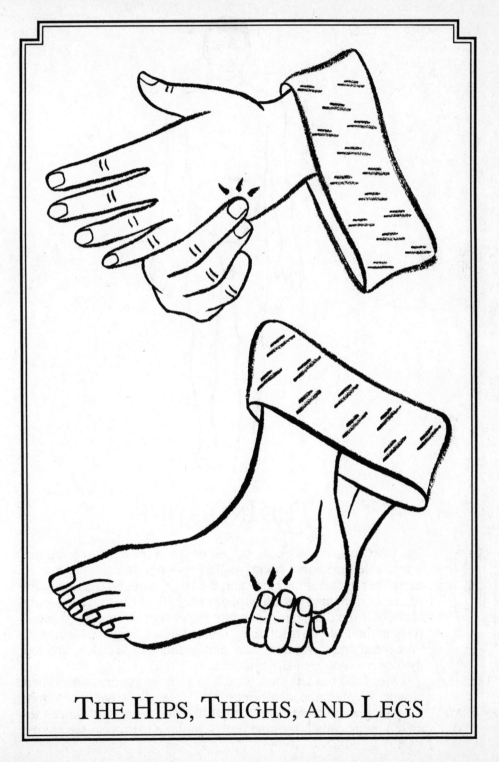

THE HIPS, THIGHS, AND LEGS

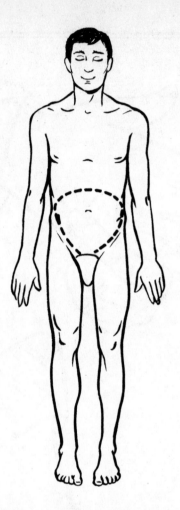

THE INTESTINE

The intestine, or bowel, the largest organ in the digestive system, is a pliable tube about twenty-eight feet long. It is usually treated as two parts, called the small and the large intestine. The small intestine is so named not because of its length but because it is only about half the diameter of the large intestine. It consists of twenty-three feet of convoluted, membrane-lined conduit, located in the central and lower abdomen, and bounded on the sides and top by the five-foot-long large intestine.

Once food has left the stomach as a thick, creamy mash called chyme, it enters the small intestine. Here, digestive juices from the pancreas and bile from the gallbladder, along with juices secreted by the small intestine itself, combine to process the chyme

LEFT HAND

into nutrient elements and water. Almost immediately, thousands of tiny, finger-shaped protrusions called villi begin to absorb fatty acids, along with important fat-soluble vitamins such as A, D, E, and K. The muscles of the small intestine undergo automatic wavelike contractions, called peristalsis, to keep the digesting chyme moving, while the nutrients, along with most of the water, are absorbed for the body's use.

Any undigested material, such as the fiber from fruits and vegetables, is passed through the ileocaecal valve into the large intestine, or colon. Since the colon is the garbage pail of the body, the ileocaecal valve is extremely important because it prevents fecal matter and bacteria from flowing back into the small intestine. As the undigested material enters the large intestine, it is pushed up the ascending colon, so named because it extends up the right side of the abdomen. The ascending colon makes a sharp left when it reaches the liver, becoming the transverse colon, which continues across the central abdomen to the left side before turning down to become the descending colon. The descending colon continues to the lower abdomen and becomes the hookshaped sigmoid colon. This joins the rectum, the last few inches of the large intestine, and leads to the anus, through which the waste is eventually emptied from the body.

The intestines suffer from an array of maladies. The entire intestinal tract is vulnerable to inflammation, which can be caused by infection, blockage, or stress. Tumors and polyps can grow in the intestines, and the colon and rectum are, next to the skin, the most common site of cancer in the Western world. Parasites such as amoebas, tapeworms, and roundworms can take up residence in the intestines, causing all kinds of problems. Two of the most common intestinal problems are constipation, sluggish or difficult bowel movements; and diarrhea, extremely liquid feces that result in sudden and frequent bowel movements.

Regulating the intestines maintains the overall health and comfort of the body, and a workout of the reflexes to the small and large intestines, as well as the ileocaecal valve, can encourage them to process nutrients into the body efficiently and empty themselves regularly of wastes. Since the intestines occupy such a large area of the abdomen, their reflex areas are easy to find on the palms and soles. On both hands, the reflex areas are the lower third of the palm, with a specific point for the ileocaecal valve located on the heel of the right palm, down from the little finger. On both feet, the intestinal reflex areas are on the sole, starting near the top of the heel and extending up to about halfway to the toes, with the point for the ileocaecal valve near the top of the right heel, down from the little toe.

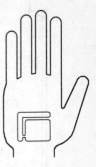

RIGHT HAND

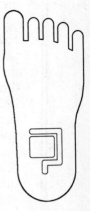

LEFT FOOT

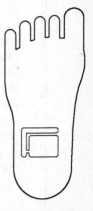

RIGHT FOOT

TECHNIQUES

When working the intestine reflex areas, be sure to cover both the right and left sides, paying particular attention to the ileocaecal reflex. Be alert for any pain or tenderness in the reflex area, as these may be a clue to some form of distress in the intestinal tract that might interfere with its functions. Work your way around the reflex area in a clockwise spiral, starting from the middle. Visualize the entire intestine and its many important digestive tasks as you work on its reflex. Breathe in as you press the reflex, and breathe out as you release the pressure.

THE HANDS — The intestine reflex areas on the hands cover a fairly large area. They are found on the lower third of the palm, and range all the way across them. The specific reflex for the ileocaecal valve is in the middle of the heel of the right palm, directly down from the crease between the ring finger and the little finger. Use your index, middle, and ring fingers to exert a firm, rolling press on the area, starting in the center and working your way to the outside perimeter in a clockwise spiral. To work the ileocaecal reflex, use your index finger to apply pressure. Start with a gentle pressure, release it slightly, then press again a little harder. You are going to cover the entire intestinal reflex area seven times, increasing your pressure each time. Do not release the pressure completely until you have finished the intestine workout.

THE FEET — On both soles, the intestine reflex areas start near the top of the heel pad, extend up a little more than halfway to the toes, and range from the inner to the outer edges. The specific reflex for the ileocaecal valve is on the right sole, near the top of the heel pad and directly down from the crease between the fourth toe and the little toe. Use your thumb to exert a firm, rolling press on the area as well as directly on the point for the ileocaecal valve. Start in the center of the area and work your way to the outside perimeter in a clockwise spiral. Begin with a gentle press, release the pressure slightly, then press again a little harder as you cover the entire intestinal reflex area seven times. Increase the pressure each time, and do not release it completely until you have finished the intestine workout.

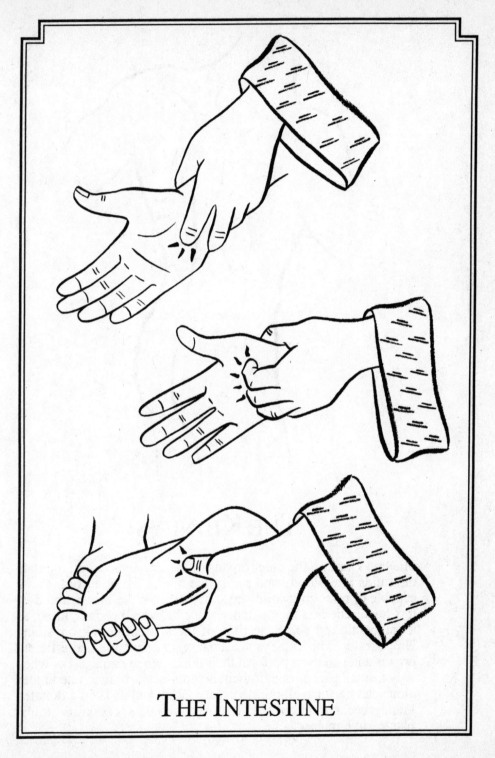

The Intestine

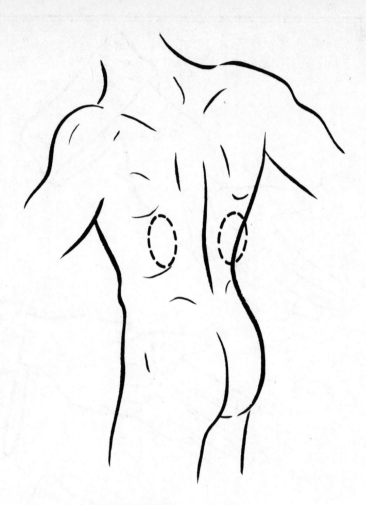

THE KIDNEYS

The two kidneys, the chief organs of the urinary system, regulate the fluids in the body and purify the blood. No other organs are capable of removing solid waste matter from the blood, and doctors have relied on the contents of the kidneys' product, urine, as a diagnostic aid since the time of the ancient Greek physician Hippocrates. The kidneys are amazingly adaptable and efficient organs and can even perform their duties when damaged or when only a small part of one of them is functional. In fact, one kidney alone can perform all the necessary tasks, and in 1954 a donated kidney became one of the first organs to be successfully transplanted in humans.

Each kidney is about the size of a fist and weighs an average of one-third of a pound. The bean-shaped organs are located behind the stomach and liver at the level of the lower-back ribs. The kidneys launder blood at the rate of about forty-eight gallons every day. When blood reaches the kidney through the renal artery, it flows into a nephron, one of the more than one million filtering units found in each healthy kidney. The nephron blocks the passage of large protein molecules and blood cells into the kidney, but takes in other fluids and small organic particles. Once in the nephron, certain enzymes, salts, sugars, and most of the water are reabsorbed by the body for other uses. The remaining fluid is combined with waste products to pass out of the kidney as urine. Every day, about one and a half to two quarts of urine are produced and excreted from the body. In this way, the kidneys control the water/salt balances in the body's cells. Thus, they regulate the blood pressure in the body and at the same time produce the hormones that trigger red blood cell production in the bone marrow.

Despite their remarkable ability to heal themselves, kidneys are subject to disease and damage from many sources. A direct blow to the kidney area can permanently destroy a number of nephrons, even the entire kidney. Nephritis, an inflammation of the kidneys, is not uncommon and can be caused by infections, by toxic materials formed in the kidneys or brought from other organs, or by any type of interference in the flow of blood to the kidneys or the flow of urine from the kidneys. One of the most common problems is kidney stones, which hospitalize one out of every thousand adults annually in the United States. Kidney stones are formed when excessive insoluble waste products such as uric acid, calcium, and oxalate are concentrated in the urine and begin to crystallize. Many of the stones are passed out of the kidney as microscopic crystals, but larger stones can be excruciatingly painful to pass. At this time, there is no permanent cure for people who form kidney stones, so prevention is the best course to take.

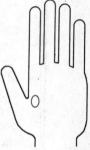

BOTH HANDS

A workout of the kidney reflexes can encourage the kidneys to flush themselves out. This can help them maintain their health by removing many of the harmful wastes that might cause nephritis. It also removes any small kidney stones and prevents the buildup of overconcentrated urine that can form these stones. The kidney reflex areas are on the palms of both hands and the soles of both feet. On the palms, the area is on the inside of the tendon to the thumb, straight down from the index finger. On the soles, the reflex area is the middle of the spongy, soft hollow of the arch, almost in the middle of the sole.

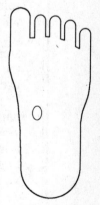

BOTH FEET

TECHNIQUES

Since there are two kidneys, there are kidney reflex areas on the palms of both hands and the soles of both feet. A general workout around the kidney reflex areas is desirable and beneficial but, for the most direct results, concentrate on the reflex area. It is also a good idea to work on both kidneys in a workout session. Visualize the kidney that you are working on and breathe in as you press the reflex, then breathe out as you release the pressure. When exerting pressure on the reflex area, note any tenderness. This may be a clue to distress in the kidney. Work the area slowly and deliberately, but be careful not to cause any real pain.

THE HANDS — To find the kidney area on both the right and left palms, place your thumb on the pad beneath your index finger. Gently slide your thumb straight down toward your wrist. Stop when you reach the inside edge of the large pad at the base of the thumb. This is the kidney reflex area. Press firmly on this area with your thumb. You are going to do this seven times. Press slowly and gently the first time, then let up slightly on the pressure, but do not stop it altogether. On subsequent presses, increase the pressure each time, pulling back between presses. Do not release the pressure completely, however, until you have finished.

THE FEET — To find the kidney area on the right and left soles of your feet, use one of your hands to flex your toes. You will then see a tendon form a ridge from the ball of your foot to the heel. Move your thumb along this tendon to a soft, spongy area about halfway between the ball and the heel, in the middle of the arch. This is the kidney reflex. Now unflex your toes and use that hand to hold them pushed toward the ball of the foot. Press firmly on the kidney reflex with the thumb of your other hand. You are going to do this seven times. The first time, press slowly and gently, release the pressure slightly, then press again, a little harder. Increase the pressure each time, pulling back between presses, but do not let up completely on the pressure until you have finished the kidney workout.

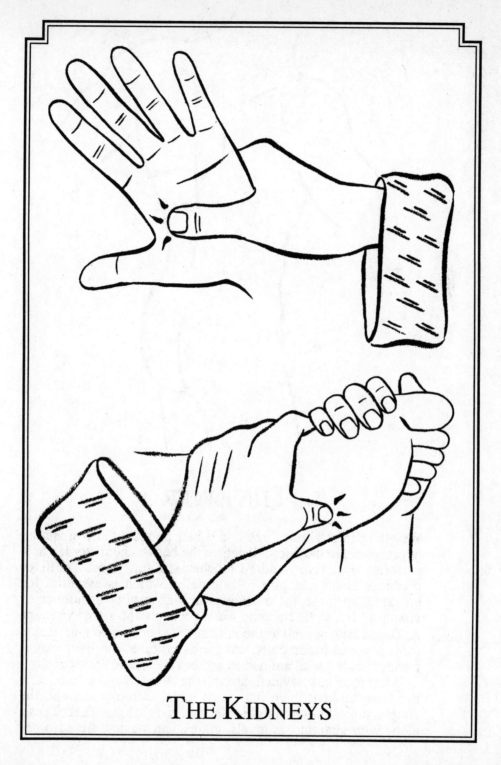

THE KIDNEYS

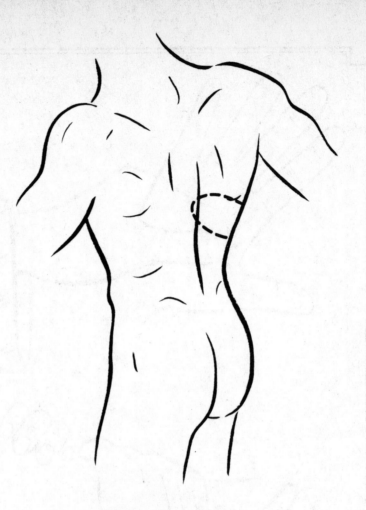

THE LIVER

Weighing in at about three and a half pounds, the liver is the largest gland in the body. It acts as the body's chemistry lab as it performs over five hundred biochemical functions. The liver produces about one pint of bile daily, which is essential for breaking up large fat molecules and absorbing a number of vitamins. It also filters toxic waste products and stores vitamins A, D, and B12, as well as the minerals copper and iron, needed to form new red blood cells. At the same time, the liver manufactures several vital antibodies and blood-clotting compounds.

After food has traveled through the stomach and intestines, it has been broken down into fatty acids, amino acids, and the simple sugar known as glucose, the body's basic fuel. These, along with vitamins, minerals, toxins, and wastes, are absorbed into the bloodstream and transported to the liver for further processing. Amino acids are turned into blood proteins such as prothrombin and fibrinogen, necessary for blood clotting, and albumin, which controls swelling by restricting the amount of fluid that flows into body tissues. Glucose is converted into glycogen and either sent on to other parts of the body or stored in the liver until needed. When a runner talks about "hitting the wall," this means that the muscles have used up all the sugar they have stored and cannot function until it is replaced. When the "fight or flight" reaction takes place, hormones from the adrenal glands incite the liver to change a large quantity of glycogen back into sugar rapidly and release it so that muscles have extra fuel for quick action. If too many carbohydrates are consumed, the liver produces an excess of glycogen and stores it in the body as fat; if the carbohydrate intake is too low, the liver breaks down stored fats and other substances to release the glucose it needs. Furthermore, the liver is a leader in the body's defense system — it converts waste into bile or into urea (a component of urine) for discharge from the body, it neutralizes poisons, and it disposes of bacteria and other foreign matter.

A healthy liver is reddish brown and located under the rib cage on the right side of the body, next to the stomach. It is able to regenerate its own tissue if damaged, unless the damage is too severe. The two most common diseases of the liver are hepatitis and cirrhosis. Hepatitis, an inflammation of the liver caused by a virus, often provokes jaundice, a yellowish tinge to the eyeballs and skin from too much bile pigment in the blood. Cirrhosis, the progressive degeneration of liver cells, is due to the presence of more foreign or toxic substances than the liver can handle. Thus, active cells are replaced by fatty scar tissue, which gives the liver a golden yellow, lumpy appearance. Cirrhosis is often due to chronic alcohol and other drug use. If caught in its early stages, cirrhosis can be treated. If not, the liver hardens, shrivels, and is unable to function, leading to death.

Clearly the liver is an indispensable organ, and working its reflex points can help it stay healthy and perform its many functions and keep the whole body in good working order. Since the liver is located on the right side of the body, the reflex areas are found only on the palm of the right hand and the sole of the right foot. On the palm, the area is just below the pads of the ring finger and the little finger, about one-third of the way between the base of the fingers and the wrist. On the sole, the area ranges from the crease between the third and fourth toes to the outer edge of the little toe, about one-third of the way between the toes and the heel.

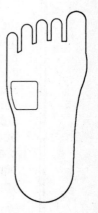

RIGHT HAND

RIGHT FOOT

TECHNIQUES

Since the liver is such a large organ, its reflex areas on the right hand and foot are also large. Work the area slowly and deliberately, and be very careful not to cause any real pain. Note any tenderness in the reflex area — this may alert you to some form of distress in the liver. Breathe in as you press the reflex, and breathe out as you release the pressure, visualizing the liver as you do so.

THE HAND — The liver reflex area is on the right palm only. It is about one-third of the way down from the bottom of the fingers toward the wrist, ranging from just below the pads at the base of the ring finger and little finger down to the top part of the pad (the "heel") at the base of the palm. The inner edge of the reflex area is directly down from the crease between the middle and ring fingers. The outer edge is down from the little finger, at the side of the hand. Grasp your hand, placing your thumb on the reflex area; use your fingers to brace it and provide resistance. With your thumb, perform a firm, rolling press on the area, slowly working the entire reflex. You are going to do this seven times. First, press and roll gently but firmly, then release the pressure a little, but do not let it up altogether. On the next rolling press, press a little harder and pull back again. Increase the pressure with each rolling press until you have finished the workout.

THE FOOT — The liver reflex area on the foot is only on the right sole. It is just below the ball of the foot and extends down to about halfway between the base of the toes and the heel pad. The inner edge is down from the crease between the third and fourth toes, and the area ranges over to the outer edge of the sole, down from the little toe. Use your thumb to perform a firm, rolling press as you move around to cover the entire reflex area. You are going to do this seven times. Press and roll gently but firmly at first, then release the pressure slightly. Increase the pressure with each subsequent rolling press, releasing it slightly between squeezes. Release the pressure completely only when you have finished the liver workout.

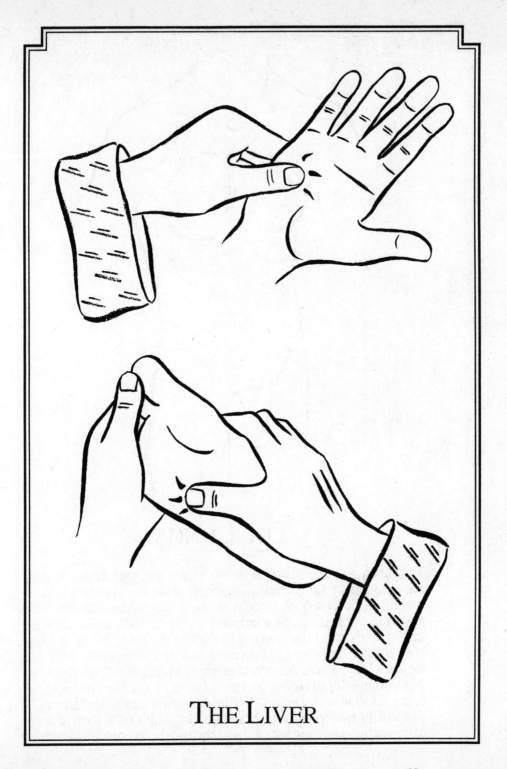

THE LIVER

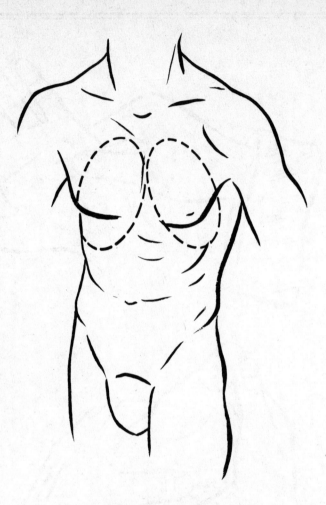

THE LUNGS

The lungs have no muscles of their own but, like bellows, they
are pumped by the surrounding chest muscles. When a person
breathes, air enters the body through the nose or mouth and
passes to the trachea, or windpipe, a tube about four inches long
that extends from the throat down into the chest. When the trachea reaches the chest, it branches into two bronchial tubes, one
for each lung. These bronchial tubes open into and form the walls
of the lungs by dividing into thousands of smaller, convoluted
branches. These branches divide again and again, to form millions of bronchioles, tiny branches the width of a human hair.
Minute clusters of air sacs are attached to the bronchioles' ends.

The lungs serve a vital role in the circulatory system. As the blood circulates through the body, it takes oxygen to the tissues for use in their metabolic processes and removes their primary waste product, carbon dioxide. The clusters of tiny air sacs exchange the carbon dioxide for oxygen. This happens at an average rate of about eighteen times every minute when the body is at rest, and increases when the body is in motion.

The lungs weigh about one pound each and are located in the chest, behind and on either side of the heart. The right lung is a little larger than the left and has three self-contained sections, while the left lung has only two lobes. Like sponges, the lungs have a crinkled surface area created by the millions of bronchioles. If the crinkles were all smoothed out, the lung's surface would spread over several hundred square feet — more than thirty times the surface area of the skin.

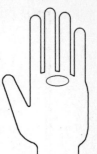

BOTH HANDS

The most common diseases of the lung are pneumonia, emphysema, cancer, abscesses, and tuberculosis. Lung abscesses and tuberculosis are both caused by bacterial infections. Pneumonia is an inflammation of the lungs usually caused by microorganisms in the lungs that trigger a buildup of fluid. When a case of pneumonia is a mild one, it is commonly referred to as "walking" pneumonia. Emphysema, often caused by environmental pollution and cigarette smoking, is the number one respiratory disease in the United States. It is a slowly developing disease in which the lungs' air sacs are destroyed and replaced with nonelastic air spaces that cannot perform the needed gas exchanges. Lung cancer, frequently caused and aggravated by smoking cigarettes, is the leading cause of cancer deaths among men and rapidly overtaking breast cancer as the leading cause of cancer deaths among women. The surgeon general of the United States estimates that over half the cases of lung cancer every year can be attributed to smoking, and the rate of lung cancer for women is rising dramatically as smoking becomes more popular among them. If diagnosed soon enough, surgery can be used to combat lung cancer, but often the disease is detected too late.

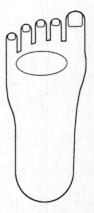

BOTH FEET

Even though the lungs have no muscles of their own, deep-breathing exercises should be performed regularly to maintain them in good working order. Stimulating the lungs through reflexology contributes to their workout and can sometimes help the lungs regenerate damaged tissues and resist infections. The lung reflex areas are found on the palms of both hands, on the pads of the middle finger and the ring finger. On the feet, the reflex areas are on the two pads that make up the balls of the feet, under the second, third, and fourth toes, and the corresponding area on the top of the feet, just above the toes.

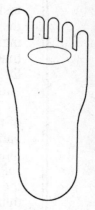

BOTH FEET

TECHNIQUES

The lungs are such large organs that their reflexes cover broad areas on the hands and feet. Work the areas for both lungs in each session, but be alert for tenderness or soreness. This could be a signal that there is some form of distress in the lungs. Take your time and work slowly and deliberately, visualizing the lungs. Breathe in as you press, and breathe out as you release the pressure.

THE HANDS — Since there are two lungs, there are lung reflex areas on the palms of both hands. The right lung is stimulated by working the right hand, the left lung by working the left. The lung areas are the pads at the base of the middle and ring fingers, and in the groove between them. Using the thumb of the opposite hand in a rolling, circular motion, press firmly as you move, and work the whole reflex area. You are going to cover the entire reflex area seven times. Begin with a slight pressure on the first press, then release the pressure a little. On the subsequent presses, continue to increase the pressure, releasing it only slightly between presses. Do not stop the pressure completely until you have finished.

THE FEET — As with the hands, stimulating the lung reflex areas on the right foot affects the right lung, while the areas on the left foot affect the left lung. On the soles of the feet, the lung reflex areas are the pads, at the base of the second, third, and fourth toes, and the grooves between the pads. Start on the area under the second toe, using your thumb in an identical way as for the hands — a circular, rolling motion as you press firmly, moving around to cover the entire reflex area. Do the entire area seven times, starting with a slight pressure and increasing it as you go. Do not stop the pressure between presses; just pull back a little until you have finished the lung workout.

The reflex areas on the top of the feet are just above the base of the second, third, and fourth toes. To work this area, put the palm of your hand against the sole for resistance, and use your index and middle fingers in place of your thumb to execute the rolling, circular pressure. Start under the fourth toe and follow the same pressing-releasing pattern that is described for the thumb.

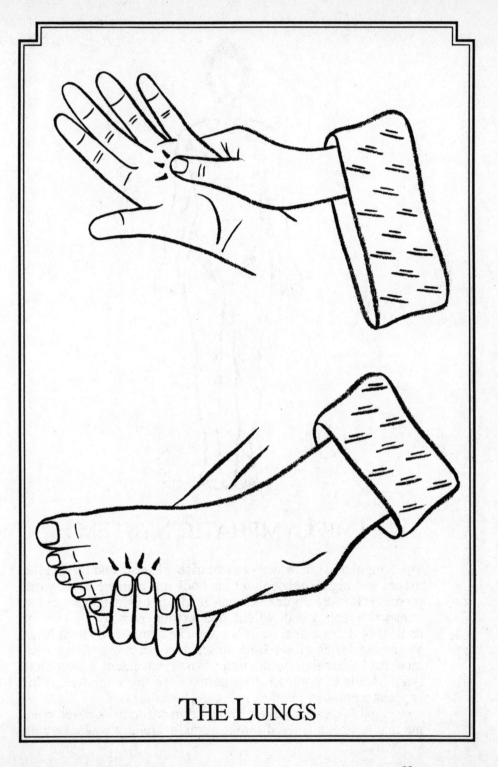

THE LUNGS

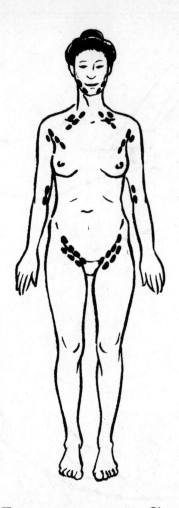

THE LYMPHATIC SYSTEM

The lymphatic system works to nourish, cleanse, and protect the tissues and organs throughout the body and remove their waste products. It is a complex network made up of small vessels that transport lymph (a bodily fluid) and provide the body with one of its lines of defense against infection. The lymphatic system is not a pumping system; it relies on muscular contractions from movement for its circulatory functions. When movement is restricted, lymph tends to pool, causing parts of the body to swell. This happens particularly in the ankles and lower legs.

Lymph, a clear or yellowish liquid, is made from blood plasma that has been filtered through small capillary walls. Lymph feeds body tissues oxygen and other nutrients while removing carbon dioxide, bacteria, and toxins or foreign matter. It is a fluid that is particularly important to the cornea of the eye, which has no blood vessels of its own and is dependent on lymph for its nutrient bath.

The lymphatic system has three main elements: the capillary network, the collecting vessels, and the lymph glands or nodes. The capillary network functions as the distribution system for lymph throughout the body. The collecting vessels carry the lymph from the capillaries and work as the lymphatic system's garbage collectors, transporting any cellular trash they have picked up to the large veins in the neck. There they empty their contents into the bloodstream for further processing. The lymph nodes are masses of tissue found at many points in the lymphatic system, particularly the groin, armpits, and neck. They are small, bean-shaped filters that help trap and remove waste products and bacteria or other infectious agents. The lymph nodes contribute lymphocytes, small white blood cells, to the lymph passing through them. There are six to seven hundred lymph nodes in the body, and each lymph node contains millions of lymphocytes that are part of the body's defense system.

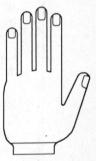

When infectious microorganisms enter the body, the lymphocytes produce antibodies to fight the invaders and neutralize their threat to the body's health. The lymph nodes can produce from ten thousand to one hundred thousand different kinds of specifically sensitized lymphocytes. In a crisis situation, some lymphocytes can generate two thousand antibodies a second. This is why, when infection is present in the body, the lymph glands swell so suddenly, producing an aching, tender feeling in the areas around them.

BOTH HANDS

Because of its role in contributing antibodies, the lymphatic system reacts and is vulnerable to many diseases, ranging from the virally caused infectious mononucleosis, or "kissing disease," to elephantiasis, a tropical disease carried by certain mosquitoes. Elephantiasis blocks the filtering actions of the lymph nodes, resulting in gross swelling of many parts of the body, especially the legs and the genitals.

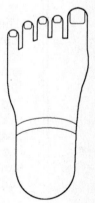

A reflexology workout of the lymphatic system can help maintain the health and disease-fighting abilities of this important member of the body's immune system. The reflex areas for the lymphatic system are on the back surface of both hands where they meet the wrists, from the outer edges under the little fingers, over to the area down from the index fingers. On the feet, the reflex areas are on the top at the bend where the feet meet the ankles, and extend from the outer ankle bones to the inner ones.

BOTH FEET

TECHNIQUES

Since the lymphatic system plays such an important role in the body's immune system, stimulating its reflex areas is beneficial at any time. Concentrating on the reflex areas will produce the most direct effects, but it is a good idea to also work other reflexes as well, particularly the kidney and liver reflexes, as these organs function as filters for removing wastes from the body. Inhale as you press the reflex, and exhale as you release the pressure. Note any tender areas in the lymphatic reflex, as they can alert you to some form of distress in the lymphatic system.

THE HANDS — The lymphatic reflex areas are on the backs of both hands, where the hands meet the wrists. The areas extend from the outer edges of the hands, directly down from the little fingers, across the wrist to just inside the inner edges, directly down from the index fingers. Wrap your hand around the wrist, placing your thumb at the base of your palm for resistance. Using your index and middle fingers in a circular, rolling motion, gently "milk" the area as you move along. Release the pressure only slightly between presses. You are going to do the entire area seven times, increasing the pressure each time. Do not, however, press too hard, as the backs of the hands are extremely sensitive and bruise easily. Be sure to work the reflex areas of both hands.

THE FEET — The reflex area for the lymphatic system can be found on the top of each foot, where the foot meets the ankle. The area extends from side to side, from the inner ankle bone to the outer ankle bone. You are going to stimulate the entire area on each foot seven times, using a technique similar to that for the hands. Wrap your hand around the ankle, approaching from the top of the foot. Start with your thumb on your inner ankle bone and your fingers on your outer ankle bone. Using your index and middle fingers in the same circular, rolling, "milking" motion, press gently as you move around the area. Increase the pressure each time, and let up on it only slightly between presses. Do not stop the pressure altogether until the lymphatic workout is completed.

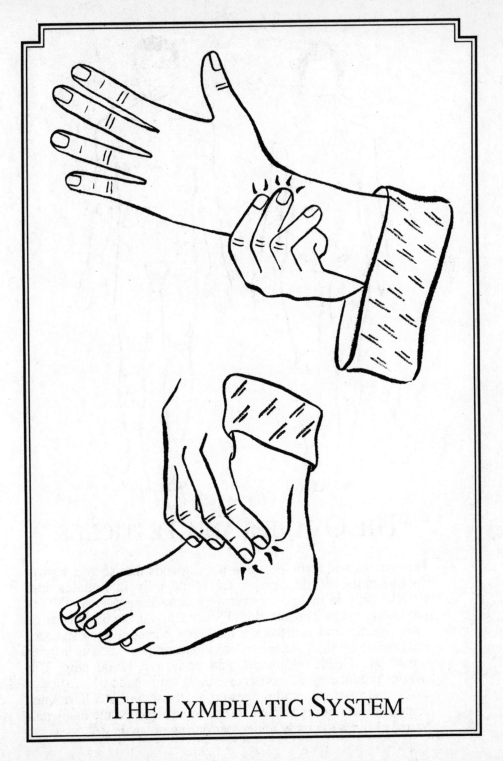

THE LYMPHATIC SYSTEM

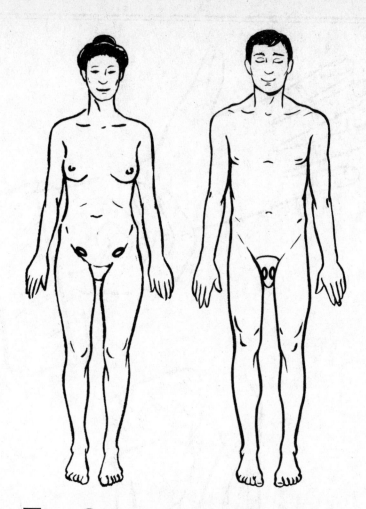

THE OVARIES AND TESTICLES

The ovaries and testicles are gonads, glands that secrete reproductive cells. While ovaries are found only in females and testicles only in males, they play corresponding parts in the reproductive cycle. The testicles produce ten to thirty billion sperm every month and secrete the male sex hormone testosterone, responsible for male secondary sex characteristics such as heavier bones, muscle development, and body and facial hair. The ovaries produce eggs, the largest single cells made by the body, and secrete estrogen and progesterone, the female sex hormones responsible for curvy bodies, menstrual cycles, and the many and varied changes the body undergoes during pregnancy.

When a little girl is born, she carries over two million eggs, or ova, in her ovaries. At puberty, three hundred thousand remain, of which about four hundred and fifty will mature and be released during her reproductive years. During these reproductive years, an ovum will mature to the size of a poppy seed and be released from the ovary about every twenty-eight days to travel through the fallopian tubes at the grand rate of one-sixteenth of an inch per hour. After about three days, it reaches the uterus where, if it has been fertilized by a sperm, it develops into a human embryo. If not fertilized, the egg is flushed out of the body along with the menstrual flow.

A man needs to produce at least four hundred million sperm each time he ejaculates if he wants to impregnate a woman. These sperm look like tiny tadpoles about one-five-hundredth of an inch long and are manufactured in the eight hundred feet of coiled tubes in the testicles. Once sperm enter a woman's vagina, they travel an average of five inches an hour in their attempt to reach the fallopian tubes and fertilize the egg. This means that the most likely time for conception is about an hour after ejaculation.

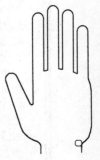

BOTH HANDS

The two ovaries, spongy masses about the size of walnuts, are in the lower abdomen, on either side of the uterus, above and behind the bladder. Ovaries are extremely sensitive to infections that usually come from other parts of the body. These include viruses that inflame glands, such as mumps; bacteria from skin and throat diseases; and venereal diseases. The formation of cysts in and on the ovaries is one of the most common ovarian problems. Other problems include the development of benign ovarian tumors, as well as malignant (cancerous) tumors that usually require the surgical removal of both the tumor and the entire ovary.

The testicles, in a thin sac of skin known as the scrotum, hang outside the body to keep the sperm cells cool. Each testicle is a soft oval gland that weighs about an ounce. Like the ovaries, the testicles are sensitive to infections traveling from other parts of the body, resulting in an inflammation known as orchitis. About one-fourth of the males who contract mumps after puberty develop orchitis. This can be prevented by immunization against mumps.

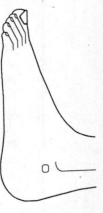

BOTH FEET

A reflexology workout stimulates the ovaries and testicles to perform their reproductive and hormonal functions, and helps maintain their health and resistance to disease. The reflex points for the ovaries in women and the testicles in men are on the sides of both feet and on the wrists. On the wrists the points are in the small indentations at the base of the outside edges of the palms. On the feet the points for the ovaries and testicles are in the pockets under the outer ankle bones.

TECHNIQUES

The reflex points for the ovaries and testicles are in the same places on the hands and feet for males as well as females. The points on a female are for ovaries, while those on males are for testicles. Visualize the ovary or testicle that you are working on and inhale as you press the reflex, then exhale as you release the pressure. When pressing on the points, note any tenderness; this will alert you to some form of distress. Be careful not to cause any real pain, but be deliberate when applying pressure.

THE HANDS — Since there are two ovaries or testicles, reflex points are located on both hands. The left reflex stimulates the left gland, while the right reflex stimulates the right, but it is a good idea to stimulate both sides rather than only one. The reflex is at the base of the palm, actually on the wrist, on the outer edge. It is in the little hollow formed between the bone at the base of the palm, straight down from the little finger, and the bone at the bottom of the arm, just at the wrist. Work on this reflex point by placing the hand palm down. Wrap your other hand around the wrist so that your thumb is on top and your index finger is on the reflex. Press gently but firmly with your index finger, then release the pressure slightly. On the next press, exert a little more pressure, then pull back again. You are going to do this seven times to each gonad reflex point, gradually increasing your pressure, with slight releases between presses. Be sure not to let up on the pressure completely until you have finished.

THE FEET — The reflex points on both feet are in the hollows under the outer ankle bones, just above the middle of each hollow. These are extremely sensitive areas, so be careful when working on them. Using a technique identical to that for the hands, you are going to stimulate each of these points seven times. Place your thumb on the hollow under the inside ankle bone for resistance and, using your index finger, press firmly on the reflex. The first time, press slowly and gently. Release the pressure slightly, then begin your next press. Increase the pressure on the subsequent presses, backing off a little between them, but do not let up on the pressure completely until the end of the ovaries and testicles workout.

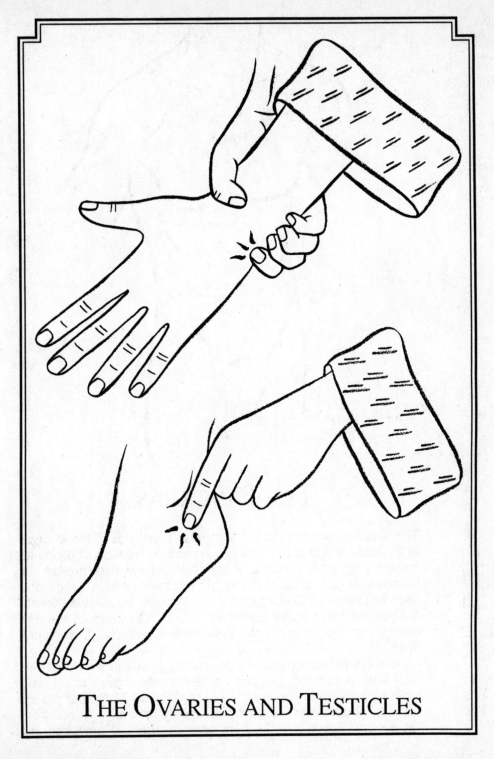

THE OVARIES AND TESTICLES

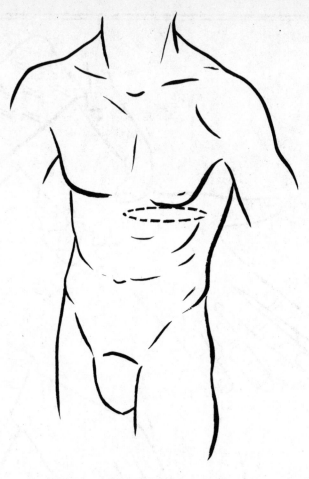

THE PANCREAS

The pancreas is the organ that controls the balance of blood sugar in the body and aids in the digestion and conversion of food into nutrients the body can use. After food has traveled through the stomach, it passes into the small intestine, which sends one chemical message to the gallbladder to release bile and another to the pancreas to release pancreatic juices. These travel through separate ducts, entering the small intestine through the same opening.

In the small intestine, the pancreatic juices break down fats into fatty acids and glycerin, proteins into amino acids, and carbohydrates into the simple sugar glucose. These are passed into the bloodstream for use or storage by the body. In addition, the pancreas produces the hormones insulin and glucagon and

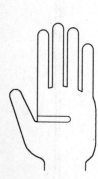

LEFT HAND

dispenses them directly into the bloodstream to control the body's blood-sugar levels. The release of these hormones is controlled by the amount of sugar present in the blood.

The secretion of insulin and glucagon makes the pancreas one of the primary regulatory organs in the body. Normally, food sugar and starch are changed into energy-rich glucose that is stored in the liver and muscles as glycogen for later use. Insulin is the key ingredient in this conversion process, while glucagon is the needed component that reconverts the glycogen back into glucose. If too much insulin is produced, a state of hypoglycemia, or low blood sugar, exists: The body is processing too much glucose out of the blood, not leaving enough in the blood for metabolic purposes, which can result in dizziness, nausea, anxiety, a feeling of faintness, and in extreme cases, convulsions and coma. Since glucose is the primary food for the brain, as well as for all the other cells in the body, the central nervous system is particularly vulnerable when hypoglycemia occurs. If the pancreas secretes too little insulin, the body cannot process carbohydrates into a usable form, resulting in diabetes mellitus, a condition that affects about four million people in the United States. The diabetic is unable to metabolize the glucose, which stays in the blood and is excreted by the kidneys directly into urine, placing a great strain on the kidneys.

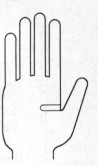

RIGHT HAND

The pancreas is about six inches long, yellow in color, and found horizontally behind the stomach, about three inches above the navel. It is a loose, soft, spongy gland with a rounded "head" on the right side, a one-inch-long "neck," and a "tail" on the left side of the body. Among the most serious pancreatic problems are pancreatitis, an inflammation often caused by alcoholism or liver and gallbladder diseases, and cystic fibrosis, a disease that produces excessive mucus which blocks ducts to and from the pancreas and can cause bile to back up into the pancreas, triggering the digestion of the pancreatic tissues themselves.

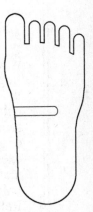

LEFT FOOT

A workout of the reflexes to the pancreas can help keep the pancreas in a sensitive state and in good working order. It may also stimulate the pancreas to produce regular amounts of pancreatic juices for digestion. The reflex areas for the neck and tail of the pancreas are primarily on the left palm, in the middle third, ranging from the ring finger to the edge of the palm under the index finger; and on the left sole, about halfway between the toes and the heel, ranging from the fourth toe to the edge of the foot under the big toe. The reflex area for the head of the pancreas is on the right palm below the index finger, about halfway between the fingers and the wrist; and on the right sole under the big toe, about halfway between the toes and the heel.

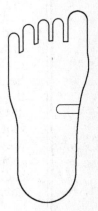

RIGHT FOOT

TECHNIQUES

Although the pancreas is one gland, its location more or less in the center of the body means that its reflex areas are on both palms and both soles. Since the greater part of the pancreas is on the left side, the reflex areas on the left hand and foot are larger than those on the right. Be sure to work the entire organ in a session. Exert a firm pressure, but be careful not to cause any pain. Tenderness in the reflex areas may indicate some form of distress in the gland. Visualize the part of the pancreas that you are working on, and inhale as you press the reflex, exhaling as you release the pressure.

THE HANDS — The pancreas reflex area on the right palm is located almost two-thirds of the way between the base of the fingers and the wrist, and extends from below the crease between the middle and the index fingers over to the edge of the hand below the index finger. On the left palm, the reflex area is in the same place, but extends from under the ring finger, across to the edge of the palm below the index finger. Using your thumb, exert a firm, rolling press on the areas. You are going to stimulate the entire reflex area on both palms seven times. Start with only a little pressure, increasing the pressure with each press. Release the pressure only slightly between presses, but do not stop it entirely until you have finished the workout.

THE FEET — The pancreas reflex area on the right sole is in the arch of the foot, about halfway between the base of the toes and the heel. It extends from the crease between the big and second toe to the inside edge of the foot. On the left sole, the pancreas reflex is in the same location, but it extends from the fourth toe over to the inside edge of the foot. Use your hand to gently hold the toes pushed toward the ball of the foot. Press firmly on the reflex areas with your thumb, using a firm, rolling press. You are going to do this seven times, using a technique identical to that for the hands. Press slowly and gently the first time, then release the pressure slightly. On the second press, exert a little more pressure, then pull back a little again. Increase the pressure each time, but do not release the pressure completely until you have finished the pancreas workout.

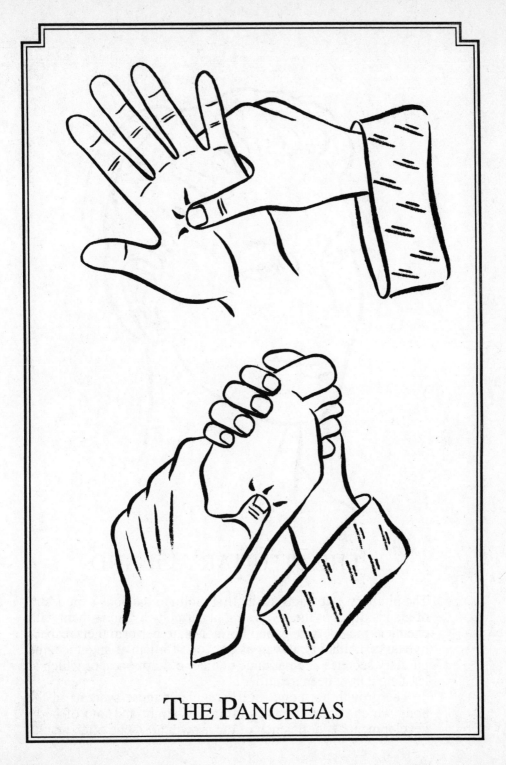

THE PANCREAS

THE PITUITARY GLAND

The pituitary gland acts as the first violin to the body's orchestra of glands. It keeps them working in harmony by cuing them with chemical messengers, called hormones, to perform their respective tasks. Although it weighs only one-fortieth of an ounce, the pituitary secretes a remarkable number of hormones, of which at least eight have been identified.

The growth hormone (hGH) regulates those systems in the body which determine such things as height and rate of body development. A deficiency of the growth hormone often results in dwarfism, which can be successfully treated with synthetic or natural hGH if treatment is started early enough. The thyroid-stimulating hormone (TSH) controls the iodine absorption in the thyroid, thereby regulating the formation and secretion of thyroid hormones. ACTH, also known as corticotropin, stimulates the adrenal glands to produce hydrocortisone, a natural form of cortisone that combats the inflammation of body tissues. ACTH is an antidiuretic hormone that manages the amount of urine that flows out of the body, as well as the amount of fluid reabsorbed by the body from the kidneys, liver, and intestines.

In sexual and reproductive matters, at least two known pituitary hormones stimulate the production of the female hormones estrogen and progesterone, which control the egg-maturation process in menstrual cycles and many of the physical developments during pregnancy. In addition, the pituitary releases the hormone that triggers milk secretion in nursing mothers. In males, it is the pituitary that instructs the testicles to produce the male hormone testosterone, which controls the male secondary-sex characteristics, such as facial and body hair growth, muscle development, and general sexual interest.

The pituitary gland is located in a small bony cavity in the center of the skull. It has two lobes separated by a fibrous membrane, one lobe of which is believed to be an ancient part of the brain. Interestingly enough, it is only in mammals that these lobes are fused together: In other life forms these lobes are two distinct parts in the body.

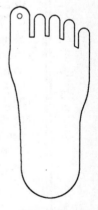

BOTH HANDS

When the pituitary gland is chronically underactive, a person will be sluggish and slow. In children, an underactive pituitary gland will often retard their mental and sexual development, as well as their growth. The normal functioning of the pituitary is affected by excessive alcohol consumption, resulting in dehydration and the consequent hangover. Also, steroids, such as those taken by athletes to increase muscle production, will affect the pituitary gland, especially in men. When the pituitary detects the presence of steroids in the bloodstream, it shuts down its own production of the hormone that triggers testosterone production. This, in turn, causes a decrease in the amount of sperm produced, along with a shrinkage in the size of the testicles.

Clearly, the role reflexology plays in stimulating the pituitary gland can be of major importance to both the mind and the body. Since the pituitary gland is almost in the center of the skull, its reflex points are present on both hands and both feet. On the hands, the reflex points are in the center of the thumb pads; while on the feet, the reflex points are found in the center of the pads on the big toes.

BOTH FEET

TECHNIQUES

The pituitary reflexes are small, specific points about the size of a sesame seed. It is difficult to stimulate them without also stimulating the surrounding points, but this is actually quite beneficial. Work the reflex points on both hands or feet, as the pituitary is located in the center of the skull and the reflex point is therefore "split" into two sides. Visualize the pituitary gland and all of its regulatory functions as you are working on its reflexes. Coordinate your workout with your breathing, so that you inhale as you press the reflex and exhale as you release the pressure. When exerting pressure on the points, note any tenderness, as this may be a clue to the presence of distress in the gland. Work slowly and deliberately, but be careful not to cause any serious discomfort.

THE HANDS — The reflex points for the pituitary gland are in the center of the pads of the thumbs. The points are actually fairly deep under the surface and require a bit of pressure to stimulate. Grasp the thumb firmly so that its thumbnail rests against the palm of your hand and your middle finger rests on the center of the thumb pad. Using a circular motion, press deeply into the pad with your index finger, then let up on the pressure slightly. You are going to do this seven times to each thumb, exerting more and more pressure on each press. Release the pressure slightly between presses, but do not let up on it altogether until you have finished.

THE FEET — The pituitary reflex points are found at the center of the pads on the big toes. Grasp the toe between your thumb and index finger and use your thumb in a circular motion to press firmly against the reflex point. Using a similar technique to that for the hands, you are going to stimulate the points on both toes seven times each. Press deeply into the pad, release the pressure slightly, then press again. Increase the pressure with each subsequent press, releasing it a bit between presses. Do not stop the pressure altogether, however, until you have finished the pituitary workout.

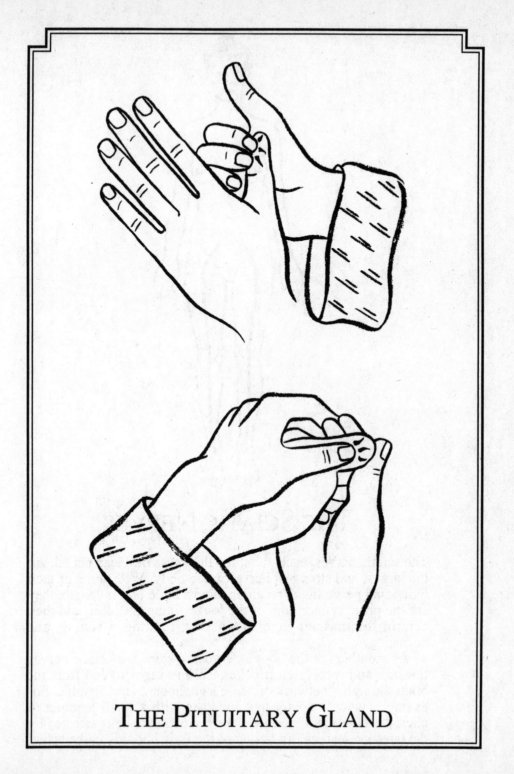

THE PITUITARY GLAND

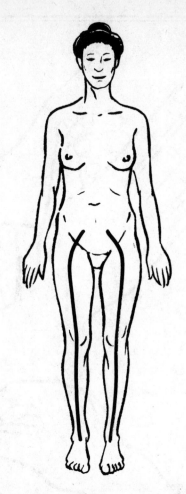

The Sciatic Nerves

The sciatic nerves, each about the thickness of a lead pencil, are the largest and strongest nerves in the body. With some of their individual nerve fibers reaching almost three feet in length, they are the primary monitors of the lower limbs and skin, and they control the muscles used in walking, running, standing, and balancing.

As members of the body's nervous system, the sciatic nerves transmit and receive electrochemical messages to and from the brain through a network of nerve switchboards in the spine. For example, when a doctor taps the knee with a small hammer to elicit the "knee-jerk" reaction, the sciatic nerve cells affected by the tap send a signal up to one of the switchboards in the spine.

Before this switchboard can pass the message on up the spine to the brain for additional analysis, it instantly transmits back a signal to the muscles in the leg to pull the knee away suddenly, making the leg jerk upward. This is actually a fast, preprogrammed emergency response in the switchboard that eliminates the extra fraction of a second needed for the brain to receive, analyze, and respond to the message — a fraction of a second that can make a real difference in the event of injury, especially an injury such as a burn. So, when the knee is tapped, what is being tested is the speed of the "switchboard" and sciatic-nerve responses — a speed that can reach three hundred and twenty-five miles an hour.

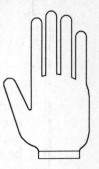

BOTH HANDS

The sciatic nerves extend from the pelvis down to the back of the femurs, or thighbones. From there, each nerve continues to just above the knee, then splits into two branches. Continuing on down the leg, the branches fan out into smaller extensions that reach to the foot and toes. Because the sciatic nerve travels just under the skin at various parts of the leg, it is particularly susceptible to injury, which often results in numbness, tingling, or pain that radiates along the nerve.

Many times, an injured or damaged spinal disc, serious constipation, a muscle spasm, or a spinal, rectal, or vaginal tumor will put pressure directly on the sciatic nerve. This causes inflammation and can lead to temporary or permanent paralysis of the leg, foot, or toes, or to a painful condition known as sciatica. A buildup of toxins such as mercury, lead, or arsenic can also trigger sciatica, as can chronic alcoholism and drug abuse. Some forms of sciatica can be eliminated by treating and eliminating their causes; others are chronic and are usually relieved through the application of heat and the use of painkillers.

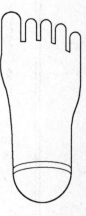

BOTH FEET

Keeping the sciatic nerves alert and in good operating condition is of primary importance in reflexology: The sciatic nerves are among the major conduits for stimulation from the reflex points on the feet to the specific organs and areas to be treated. These nerves respond well to a workout themselves, and stimulating their reflex points may alleviate some attacks of sciatica. In addition, working the sciatic nerves can improve the overall condition of the legs, knees, ankles, feet, and toes, making the sciatic reflexes very important indeed. Since there are sciatic nerves in both legs, the reflex areas are found on both hands and both feet. On the hands, the reflex areas are on the inside of the wrists, extending from one edge to the other. On the feet, the reflex areas are under and behind the inner and outer ankle bones, as well as almost in the center of the heel pads, extending all the way across the width of the heels to the edges of the feet.

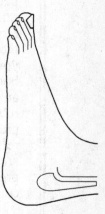

BOTH FEET

TECHNIQUES

Since the sciatic nerves are so very important to the general applications of reflexology, a regular workout of their reflexes is an excellent idea. Rather than concentrating on just one side of the body, the reflexes of both the left and right sciatic nerves should be stimulated. Be very conscious of tenderness or soreness in the reflex areas. This may be a clue to distress in the sciatic nerves. Use a firm pressure, but be careful not to cause any real pain: In cases of sciatica, there is already excruciating pain present, so work to relieve it, not increase it. Visualize the sciatic nerve that you are working on, inhale as you press the reflex, and exhale as you release the pressure.

THE HANDS — The sciatic reflex areas on the hands are found on the inside of the wrists and extend from edge to edge. Using the tip of your thumb in a firm, almost digging motion, press gently on the reflex area, releasing the pressure slightly, then pressing again just a little harder. You are going to do this seven times, covering the entire sciatic reflex area. Each time you press, exert a little more pressure than on the previous press. Release the pressure only a little between presses, but do not stop it completely until you have finished.

THE FEET — The sciatic reflex areas on the feet are in three places: the strips running underneath and behind the outer and inner ankle bones, and the narrow bands in the middle of the heel pads that extend horizontally from edge to edge. On the heel reflex area, use the tip of your thumb in a firm, almost digging motion to push. For the ankle area, grasp the foot from behind the ankle so that your thumb is next to the outer ankle bone and your index finger and middle finger are next to the inner ankle bone. Do not dig into this area as you would for the heel — the ankle areas are extremely sensitive reflexes. Press firmly, then release the pressure slightly. Push a little harder on the next press, again releasing the pressure just a little. As with the sciatic reflex areas on the hands, you are going to treat all the reflex areas on each foot seven times. Increase the pressure with each press, and release it a little between presses, but do not stop it completely until the sciatic workout is finished.

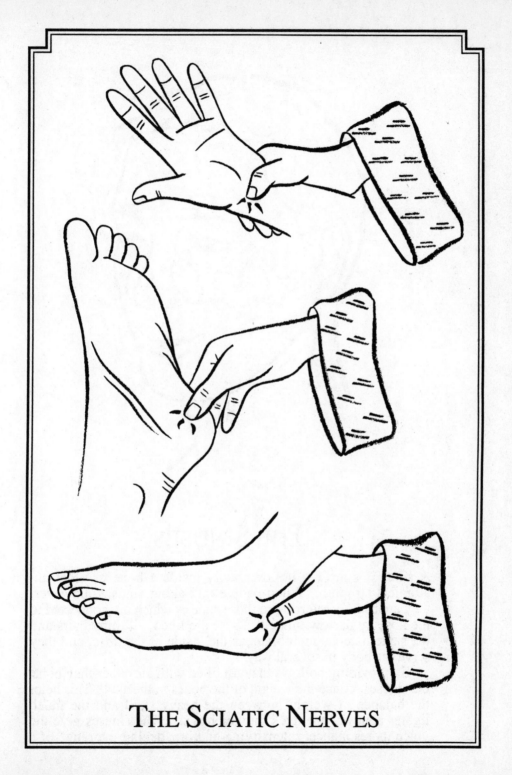

THE SCIATIC NERVES

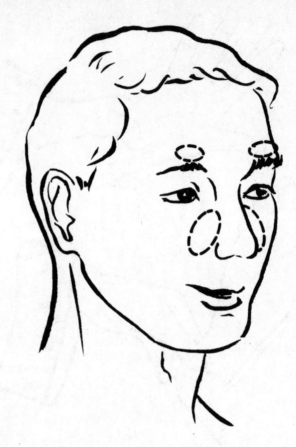

THE SINUSES

A sinus is simply a hollow cavity inside a bone or other anatomical structure. When people talk about sinuses, however, they are usually referring to those sinuses which are connected to the nose by narrow tunnels. These are lined with tiny hairs and the same mucous membrane as the inside of the nose, and they serve the body in several ways.

By providing hollows that are filled with air rather than bone, the sinuses reduce the weight of the bones in the skull. This helps the balance of weight between the heavy skull and the much lighter bones of the neck on which it sits. The sinuses give the voice its resonance, intensifying and broadening the range of a speaker's or singer's voice. The mucous membranes in the sinuses secrete mucus that, along with the waving motions of the little hairs, collects and blocks the dust, germs, and other unwelcome foreign particles which enter the body through the nose. This prevents these from entering the lungs, making the sinuses another of the body's front lines of defense against invasion and infection.

There are four basic pairs of sinuses related to the nose. The sphenoid sinuses are two irregularly shaped cavities in the back of the head. The frontal sinuses are above the eyes on the forehead and, when inflamed, are the ones most often responsible for a sinus headache. Just beneath them, but behind the eyes and nose, are the ethmoid sinuses, which open directly into the cavities of the nose. These are also contributors to the sinus headache. Under the eyes, extending down toward the upper jaw, are the maxillary sinuses, the ones primarily affected by tooth and gum problems.

Because of their connection to the nasal passages, the sinuses are vulnerable to many things. Pollens that trigger hay fever and other allergies can irritate the membranes of the sinuses and cause them to swell. Viruses that cause the common cold and flu can settle in the sinuses, triggering uncomfortable symptoms and exposing the throat and ears to infection. Polluted air often irritates the sinuses and makes breathing difficult; and germs from infections in the mouth can travel up to the sinuses and infect their mucous membranes. When any of these irritants are present, the mucous membranes lining the sinuses become inflamed and the sinuses may fill with pus. This condition is called sinusitis, and usually manifests itself as a headache, frequently accompanied by a yellowish or greenish discharge that seeps down into the nose and throat.

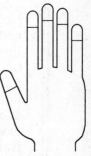

BOTH HANDS

A reflexology workout of the sinuses achieves two aims. The first is preventative; stimulation can help keep the mucous membranes of the sinuses healthy and can encourage them to drain accumulated debris regularly. The second is remedial; reflexology has been known to alleviate cases of sinusitis, unblocking clogged air passages and relieving the accompanying headaches.

The reflex areas for the sinuses are on both hands and both feet. Those on the left hand and foot correspond to the left sinuses, while those on the right hand and foot stimulate the right sinuses. On the hands, the sinus reflex areas are the top joints and knuckles of the thumbs and fingers, including the pads, tips, sides, and areas of and below the nails. On the feet, the areas are the top joints and knuckles of the toes and, as with the hands, also include the sides, tips, pads, tops, and nails.

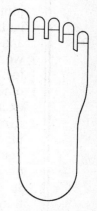

BOTH FEET

...ile a general treatment of the reflexes near the sinus reflex areas is beneficial, working on the specific reflexes will yield the most direct results. Take your time and cover all the reflex areas, working them slowly and deliberately. Treat both the right and left sinus areas in a session rather than concentrating on just one side, even if there seem to be problems on only one side. Visualize the sinuses that you are working on, and inhale as you press the reflex, exhaling as you release the pressure. Be careful not to cause any real pain as you work, and be alert for any tender areas. These are clues to some form of distress in the sinuses and can alert you in time to head off potential problems.

THE HANDS — The sinus reflex areas on both hands are the top joints and knuckles of the thumbs and fingers. These include the entire joint, the pads, tips, sides, nails, and areas under the nails. Grasp the top joint between your thumb, index finger, and middle finger and use a firm, rolling, pressing motion. Set up a sequence that starts with the thumb, then goes on to each of the other fingers. Press gently the first time you go through the sequence, then press a little harder on the next sequence. Increase the pressure with each new sequence until you have pressed the thumb and each finger seven times. After finishing the last sequence, give the thumb and each finger three or four light clockwise and counterclockwise twisting motions to finish off.

THE FEET — The sinus reflex areas on both feet are the top joints and knuckles of the toes, including the pads, tips, sides, nails, and areas under the nails. For support, first place the index and middle fingers of one hand on the nail of the toe to be worked. Then put the thumb of your other hand on the pad of the toe, and use the index and middle fingers of this hand to press the other fingers against the toe. This gives you enough leverage to exert the pressure you need to stimulate the reflex area. Use a firm, rolling, pressing motion. In a sequence that starts with the big toe, then goes on to each of the other toes, press gently with your fingers and thumb. Increase the pressure with each new sequence until all the toes have been worked seven times. After all seven sequences have been done, finish off each toe by twisting it lightly three or four times in a clockwise and counterclockwise motion.

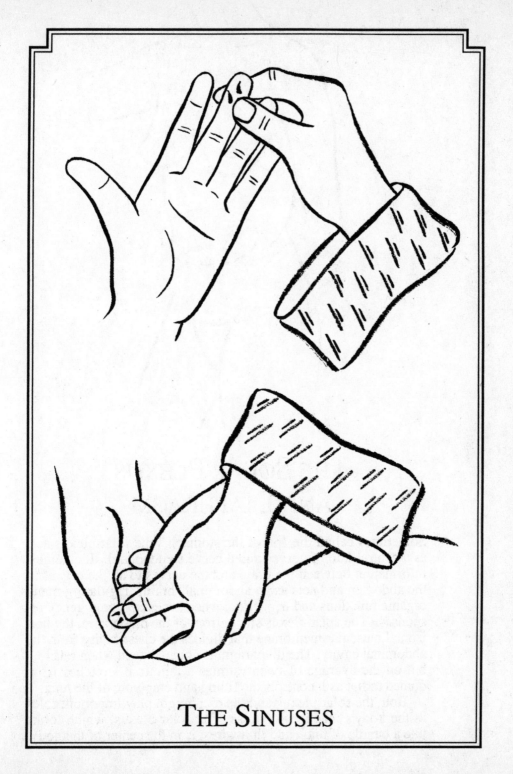

THE SINUSES

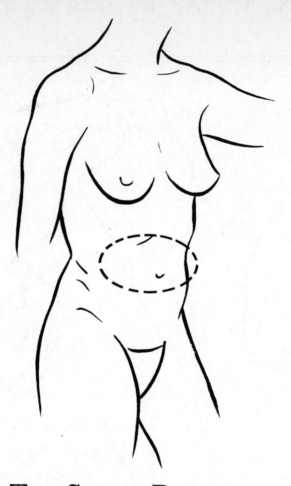

THE SOLAR PLEXUS
AND DIAPHRAGM

Sometimes called the "pit of the stomach," the solar plexus acts as a central hub of nerves and a nerve switchboard. It channels information between the brain and the nerves to all the organs in the abdomen and acts as an abdominal "brain," regulating many organic functions and triggering, when necessary, emergency responses. The solar plexus sits in front of the diaphragm, the horizontal muscular membrane that divides the chest cavity from the abdominal cavity. The diaphragm is dome-shaped when relaxed, but on the average of twenty times a minute it stretches from domed to flat as it controls the filling and emptying of the lungs.

Both the solar plexus and the diaphragm play important roles in the body's reaction to stress. The solar plexus, which looks like a bundle of thick and thin wires, is in the center of the body, behind and above the stomach and between the adrenal glands. After receiving information from its many nerves, the solar plexus determines which muscles and organs in the abdomen should tense or relax, and it conveys "fight-or-flight" instructions from the brain to the adrenal glands. It also functions as the "manager" of the abdomen. Among many other supervising duties, it passes on reminders to the stomach and intestines to keep the food processing moving along, to the liver to produce bile and filter toxins, and to the kidneys to remove wastes.

The diaphragm is a muscle that extends laterally across the middle of the body from the bottom of the breastbone back to the spine. It is very important to the process of breathing, and this influences a range of functions, from how quickly muscles respond in an emergency to how deeply the body sleeps at night. The diaphragm is a muscle and thus it is subject to tears and spasms. Sometimes, due to an injury or developmental defect, the diaphragm tears and the stomach protrudes up into the chest cavity. This is known as a hiatal hernia, which can be treated surgically or, in less severe cases, can heal itself if it is not aggravated by heavy, difficult-to-digest meals.

When the diaphragm suffers an involuntary spasm, it closes the opening between the vocal cords when a breath is taken, blocking the intake of air. This produces a series of sharp, gasping breaths known as hiccups or hiccoughs. There are many things that trigger these spasms, such as eating too quickly, gulping foods or liquids that are too hot, and attacks of anxiety or other forms of psychological stress. A high concentration of carbon dioxide in the blood helps get rid of hiccups by forcing the diaphragm to relax. This can be accomplished by holding one's breath for as long as possible and by breathing into a paper (not plastic) bag, thereby taking carbon dioxide back into the body. Other remedies, such as drinking a glass of water quickly or eating a teaspoon of granulated sugar, force the vocal cords apart, allowing air to enter and stop the spasm.

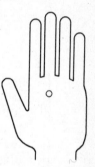

BOTH HANDS

The solar plexus and diaphragm reflexes are of primary importance in reflexology because they are critical in the processes of stress and relaxation. Since so many problems in the body are stress related, every workout session, regardless of what other parts are being stimulated, should include working these reflexes. Their location is, effectively, on top of each other, so stimulating the solar plexus reflexes on the palms and soles automatically stimulates the diaphragm reflexes. These points are in the center of the palms of both hands, just below the pads at the base of the middle fingers, and on the soles of both feet, just below the two large pads that make up the balls of the feet.

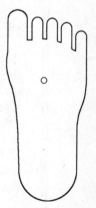

BOTH FEET

TECHNIQUES

It is an excellent idea to stimulate the solar plexus and diaphragm reflexes in every session, as these reflexes are intricately involved in stress control and relaxation. Even in situations where there is little or no time for a full treatment of specific parts of the body, the relaxation alone produced by stimulating the solar plexus and diaphragm will trigger general beneficial responses. While there is only one solar plexus and one diaphragm in the body, they are both centrally located and cover a broad area, so be sure to work the areas on both the right and left palms or soles. Visualize the solar plexus and the diaphragm as you stimulate their reflexes; inhale as you press the reflex, and exhale as you release the pressure.

THE HANDS — The solar plexus and diaphragm reflexes are in the same location and they are stimulated together. The reflex points are on the palms of both hands, just beneath the pads of the middle fingers. For the best leverage, approach the palm to be treated from the index-finger edge rather than the little-finger edge. Place your thumb firmly on the point. You will notice that the fingers on the hand being treated try to curl: Force them to straighten, as this exposes the reflex for easier stimulation. Press your thumb into the point and use the movement of your entire hand and wrist to rotate the thumb. Let up a little on the pressure, then repeat the motion again, pressing a little harder. You are going to do this seven times to each palm, increasing the pressure a little each time. Do not let up on the pressure completely until you have finished.

THE FEET — The reflex points for the solar plexus and diaphragm are on the soles of both feet, in the center, just below the balls of the feet. Place your thumb firmly on the reflex and use your other hand to flex the toes, rather than letting them curl. Use your entire hand and wrist to press and rotate the thumb seven times on each sole. Release the pressure a little, then repeat the motion again, pressing a bit harder. Increase the pressure a little each time and release it only slightly in between presses. Do not stop the pressure completely until the solar plexus and diaphragm workout is completed.

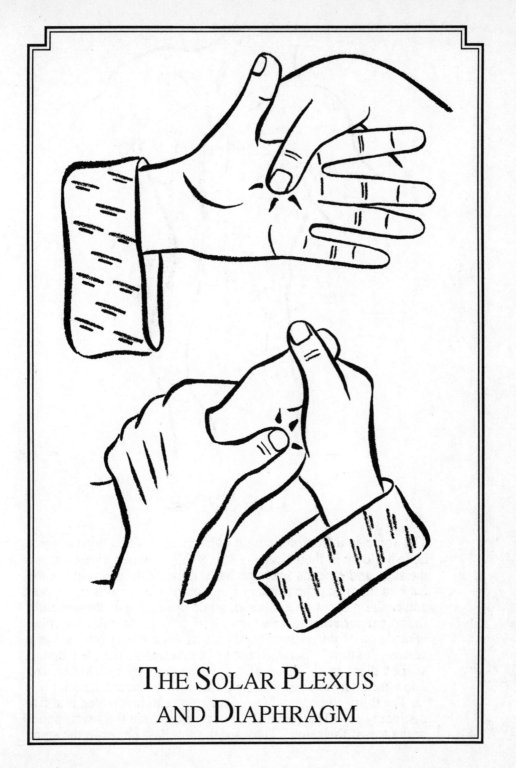

THE SOLAR PLEXUS
AND DIAPHRAGM

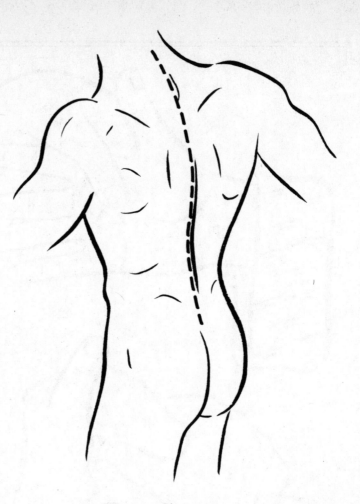

THE SPINE

The spine is a flexible, single column of stacked bones which have hollows in their centers. It is S shaped when viewed from the side, and extends from the base of the skull, down along the back to the hips. The primary function of the spine is to support and cushion the skull and torso, while protecting and channeling the spinal cord that travels through its center. At birth, the spine is made up of thirty-three bones called vertebrae (from the Latin *vertere,* "to turn"). Between each of the vertebrae there are donut-shaped discs made of cartilage. These discs absorb shock and allow the spine to twist and bend smoothly without friction.

The thirty-three vertebrae of the spine can be divided into five distinct types. The cervical, or neck, bones are the seven bones at the top of the stack. They are the smallest bones in the spine and directly support the skull and give the head its movement. The cervical vertebrae are stacked on top of twelve larger-sized dorsal vertebrae, to which the ribs are connected. Beneath these twelve dorsals are the five lumbar, or loin, bones, the largest in the spine; and under them are the five sacral and four coccygeal vertebrae. These last two groups are unusual in that the bones in them are usually fused together in adulthood. The five sacral bones of the lower spine form a single triangular bone called the sacrum, or "sacred bone," so named because in ancient times it was believed to house the soul. The four coccygeal bones also form one unit called the tailbone, or coccyx (from the word for "cuckoo," because of its shape like a cuckoo's beak). The spine is connected just above the tailbone to each hipbone, or ilium, by the sacroiliac.

The spinal cord, extending down the middle of the spine, is a direct extension of the central nervous system from the brain. It is about eighteen inches long in an adult, about as thick as a little finger, and gives off thirty-one pairs of nerves between the vertebrae. The spinal cord is H shaped when viewed in cross section and is made up of gray matter such as is found in the brain, along with white nerve fibers that relay information to and from the brain. With over ten billion nerve cells, about half the nerve cells of the body, the spinal cord acts as the body's switchboard. It controls such things as the reflexive reactions that cause a hand to pull away from a hot stove or a knee to jerk when tapped by a hammer. These are emergency reactions triggered by information that comes directly from the spinal cord rather than the brain.

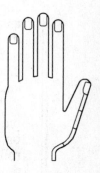

BOTH HANDS

The problems affecting the spine itself are many. The vertebrae are subject to fractures, to deviations in curvature, and to dislocations. The discs between the vertebrae can be ruptured or dislocated, often putting painful pressure on the spinal cord or other nerves. In the spinal cord, problems include spinal meningitis, an inflammation of the membranes around the spinal cord caused by infection; polio, a viral infection that destroys the nerve roots controlling motor functions; and multiple sclerosis, a disease in which the sheath surrounding the nerves is destroyed and replaced by scar tissue, blocking nervous functions.

A workout of the spine reflex areas helps keep the spine flexible and stimulates the spinal cord, affecting the alertness and health of all the nerves that radiate from this switchboard. Since the spine is in the middle of the body, its reflex areas are on both hands and both feet. On the hands, the areas extend along the outer edges of the thumbs down onto the wrists. On the feet, the spinal reflex areas are on the inner edges from the big toe, down through the arches, to the base of the heels.

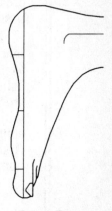

BOTH FEET

TECHNIQUES

The spine and spinal cord are located on the midline of the body, so their reflexes are divided between the right and left hands and feet. Since the spine and spinal cord are so important to the overall structure and nervous responses of the body, be sure to work the reflexes on both sides, rather than just concentrating on one. The reflex areas reflect different sections of the spine. The edges of the thumb and big-toe pads are the reflex areas for the neck. The edges below this are the reflexes for the dorsal area, followed by the reflexes for the lumbar section. The wrist and heel edges are the reflexes for the sacrum and tailbone. Visualize the area of the spine that you are working on. Breathe in as you press the reflex, and breathe out as you ease the pressure. Pay attention to any tenderness in the spine reflex areas, as this can be a clue to problems that might be developing. Work the area slowly and deliberately, but be careful not to cause any pain or bruising.

THE HANDS — The spine reflexes are along the edges of the hands and extend from just below the top of the thumbs down onto the wrists. Use your thumb to work the area with a firm, rolling press, starting on the edge of the thumbnail and working down the side of the hand in one pass. You are going to cover the entire spine reflex area seven times, starting with a gentle pressure on the first pass. On the next pass down the reflex area, increase the pressure, and keep increasing it on all subsequent passes until you have finished the spine workout.

THE FEET — On the feet, the spine reflexes are along the inner edges and extend from the middle of the big toenails down to the bottom edges of the heels. Work the area with your thumb, using a firm, rolling press. Start on the edge of the toenail and work down to the bottom of the heel in one pass. As you did with the reflexes on the hands, you are going to work the entire spine reflex area seven times. Begin with a gentle pressure on the first pass, increasing it on subsequent passes until you have completed the spine workout.

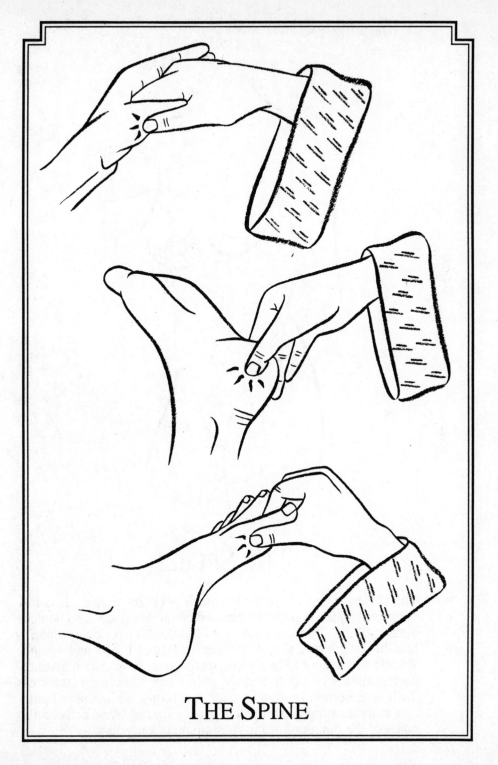

THE SPINE

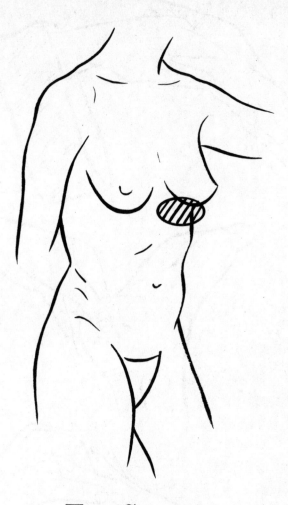

THE SPLEEN

The spleen is one of the body's most peculiar organs. It is insensitive to pain and can be removed completely or transplanted outside of the abdominal cavity with little ill effect on a person's health. This large, purplish organ is full of blood and lymph vessels and seems to be two organs in one, having two distinct parts, called white pulp and red pulp. The white pulp concerns itself with certain immunological operations, while the red pulp acts as a cleansing and recycling agency for red blood cells. Still, many of the functions of the spleen remain a mystery.

What little is known about the spleen can be simply summarized. It filters and stores blood, releasing it as needed to maintain the blood volume in the body's circulatory system. The spleen also breaks down old red blood cells to store and replenish hemoglobin, the "iron" needed in blood to prevent anemic conditions, and is involved in the metabolic processes that yield uric acid, one of the components of urine. The spleen is also believed to be active in the digestive processes, since it enlarges slightly during the digestion of food and is found to be quite small in starving people. Acting in the same role as a lymph node, the spleen filters out impurities and toxins in the lymph fluid, while it also manufactures lymphocytes, the small white blood cells that are so important in the body's immune and defense systems. The spleen, however, is not an indispensable organ and, in cases where it has been removed surgically, its functions seems to be adequately duplicated in the liver, bone marrow, and lymph nodes.

The average healthy spleen is about five inches long, three inches wide, and one and a half inches thick. It weighs about seven ounces and can be found in the lower left side of the ribcage, between the back of the stomach and the diaphragm. The spleen does not have any ducts to other organs but, instead, sends out its secretions directly in the blood and lymph, making it the largest ductless gland in the body.

The spleen does not seem to have any specific disorders related to it. Instead, it reacts to direct injuries and to complications from infections and diseases in other parts of the body, such as malaria, some forms of cancer and leukemia, and an assortment of viral infections. When these conditions are present, the spleen usually becomes enlarged — in some cases, it has been known to balloon up to thirty times its original size. If the conditions causing the enlarged spleen cannot be successfully treated, the spleen is often removed, seemingly with no ill effects, although people without spleens are sometimes more vulnerable to infectious diseases and anemia.

While in many ways the spleen seems to be a superficial organ, it is nonetheless a part of a healthily functioning body. A reflexology workout of the spleen can help to keep it healthy, and thus increase the body's resistance to infection and disease. Since the spleen is on the left side of the body, its reflex areas are only on the left palm and left sole. On the left palm, the reflex point is about halfway between the base of the fingers and the wrist, under the little finger. On the left sole, the reflex area is about halfway between the toes and the heel, under the fourth and little toes.

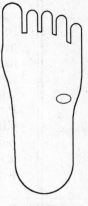

LEFT HAND

LEFT FOOT

103

TECHNIQUES

Because the spleen is found on the left side of the body, its reflex areas appear only on the left palm and left sole. Exert a firm and deliberate pressure when you stimulate the reflex, but be careful not to cause any real discomfort or bruise the tissues on the hand or foot. Note any tenderness in the spleen reflex area, as it may indicate some form of distress in the gland that might inhibit the performance of its tasks. While you are working on its reflex, visualize the spleen and imagine its disease-fighting, blood-cleansing, and hemoglobin-recycling functions. Carefully coordinate your breathing with your workout, so that you inhale as you press the reflex and exhale as you release the pressure.

THE HAND — The spleen reflex area on the hand is on the left palm, located just beneath the halfway point between the base of the fingers and the wrist, under the little finger. You are going to stimulate the spleen reflex area on the palm seven times, using your thumb to exert a firm, rolling press on the area. Start off with only a little pressure, then let up slightly, but do not release the pressure altogether. Increase the pressure with each subsequent press, releasing it a little between the presses. Be sure not to stop the pressure entirely until you have finished the spleen workout.

THE FOOT — The spleen reflex area on the foot is on the left sole, just about halfway between the base of the toes and the back of the heel. It extends from the crease between the third and fourth toes over to the edge of the foot under the little toe. You are going to stimulate the spleen reflex seven time, using a technique just like that for the hands. Use one hand to hold all the toes pushed toward the ball of the foot. Press on the reflex area with the thumb of your other hand, using a firm, rolling press. Press slowly and gently the first time, then release the pressure slightly. On the second press, exert a little more pressure, then pull back a little again. Increase the pressure each time, but do not let up on it completely until you have completed the spleen workout.

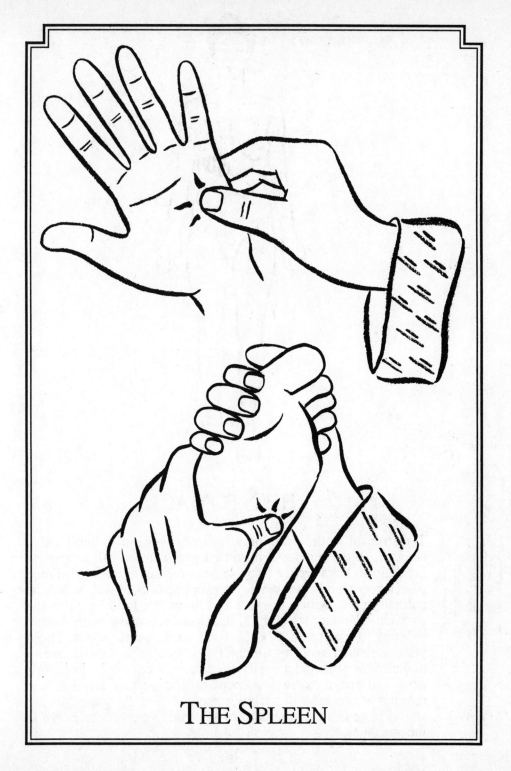

THE SPLEEN

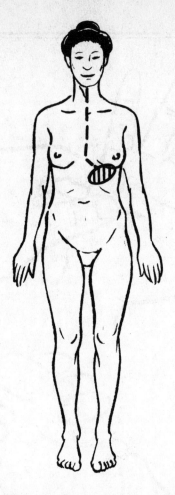

THE STOMACH

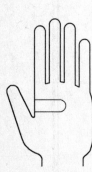

LEFT HAND

The stomach is the principal organ of digestion. When food is chewed, saliva moistens it and enzymes in the saliva start to break down the starches into usable components. The food then passes down a tube known as the esophagus to a valve called the cardiac valve, which opens and allows the food to enter the stomach. The muscles of the stomach contract about every twenty seconds to mash and mix the food with gastric juices. These juices, secreted by thirty-five million glands in the mucous membrane of the stomach, consist of acids, particularly hydrochloric acid, and enzymes, such as pepsin for digesting proteins and rennin for breaking down milk products. While some fats are also digested in the stomach, most of them are broken down in the intestines.

Interestingly enough, with the exceptions of water and alcohol, the stomach is not directly involved in the body's nutrient-absorption processes. Instead, once the food has been turned into a thick, creamy mash called chyme, the stomach ejects it in spurts through the pyloric valve into the duodenum, or small intestine, for further processing and absorption into the body. About three or four hours after the food has first entered it, the stomach is empty and ready for the next batch. When the empty stomach contracts, "hunger pangs" and rumbles are the result.

The stomach is a lopsided, bean-shaped sac, larger at its upper end than at its lower end. It sits mostly on the left side of the body, under the diaphragm and above the intestines. It changes size constantly, depending on how much food it is processing, and can usually hold up to two quarts at a time. The stomach is subject to uncomfortable spasms of either of its valves, to nausea from irritated nerve endings, and to bloating from gas.

The most common serious disorders of the stomach are gastritis and peptic ulcers. Gastritis, the inflammation of the stomach's lining, takes three forms. Acute gastritis is most often caused by food poisoning, infection, or excessively rich and fatty foods. Chronic gastritis is caused by alcoholism, vitamin deficiencies, or stress. Toxic gastritis comes as the result of swallowing poisons or corrosive substances. Peptic ulcers are caused by erosions in the mucous lining of the stomach. This allows the hydrochloric acid and other digestive juices to come in direct contact with the stomach walls, burning and dissolving them. Exactly what causes this condition is not clearly understood, but stress is considered to be one of its primary triggers.

Because the stomach is subjected to so much abuse in everyday life — ranging from inadequately chewed food to knotting tension — the role of reflexology is one of regulation and relaxation. A workout of the stomach reflexes encourages the stomach to function efficiently while maintaining the health of its muscles, its glands, and the mucous membrane lining it. Since the stomach is primarily on the left side of the body, the reflex areas on the left palm and sole are larger than those on the right. On the left palm, the reflex area is just below the pads under the ring finger, middle finger, and index finger. On the right palm, the reflex area is in the same place, but only under the index finger. On the left sole, the stomach reflex area is from about one-fourth of the way down to about one-half of the way between the toes and the heel, and ranges from directly below the crease between the third and fourth toes, over to the inner edge of the foot. The reflex is in the same area on the right sole, but only extends under the big toe.

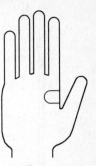

RIGHT HAND

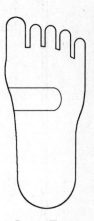

LEFT FOOT

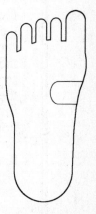

RIGHT FOOT

TECHNIQUES

The stomach reflex area on the left hand and foot is a fairly broad area, while on the right it is much smaller. This corresponds to the proportions of the stomach that are on the left and right sides of the body. While the stomach reflexes are primarily on the left palm and sole, do not neglect to work on the reflexes on the right palm and sole. Visualize the stomach as you stimulate its reflexes, inhaling as you press the reflex and exhaling as you release the pressure. Be sure to note any soreness in the reflex area. This may give you a clue to distress in the stomach.

THE HANDS — The stomach reflex extends across the middle of the left palm, just below the pads under the ring finger, middle finger, and index finger. On the right palm, the reflex area is in the same place, but only under the index finger. Use your thumb to exert a circular, rolling press. You are going to cover the entire reflex area on each hand seven times. Start with a light, rolling press, letting up the pressure slightly but not releasing it altogether. Increase the pressure on subsequent presses, but do not stop the pressure altogether until you have finished.

THE FEET — To find the stomach reflex area on the left sole, mentally divide the sole into quarters between the toes and the heel. The reflex area is in the second quarter down from the toes, below the ball of the foot, and extends from the edge of the foot under the big toe over to directly below the crease between the third toe and the fourth toe. You will find the area to be in the same place on the right sole, but extending only from the edge of the foot over to directly below the crease between the big and second toes. You are going to use a technique identical to that for the hands, as you cover the entire reflex area on each foot seven times. Press firmly with your thumb in a circular, rolling motion. Let up on the pressure a little. Increase the pressure every time you press, but do not let up on it completely until you have finished the stomach workout.

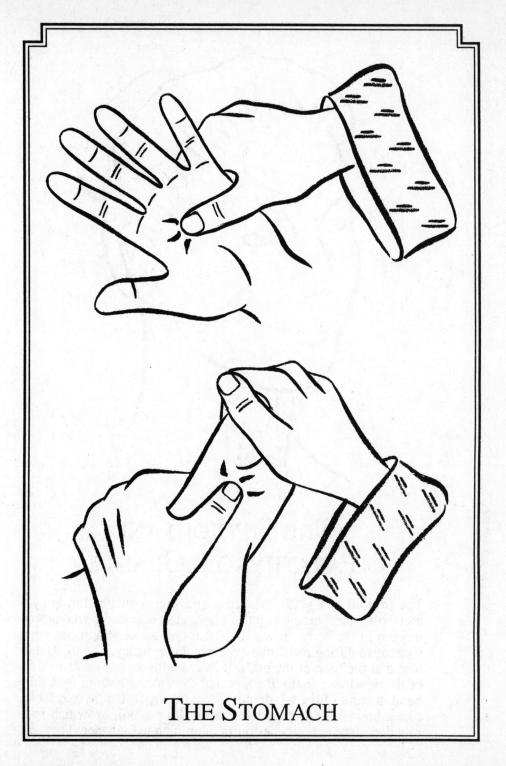

THE STOMACH

The Thyroid and Parathyroid Glands

The thyroid is a yellowish red gland that regulates the body's metabolic rates, monitors pulse rates, and controls the amounts of oxygen in the body. It weighs about one ounce and, in women, it enlarges during menstrual cycles and pregnancy. The thyroid is found at the base of the neck. It has two lobes, one on each side of the windpipe, that are connected toward the bottom by a thin band in front of the windpipe. From the front, the thyroid looks like a bow tie. The parathyroids are four small, brownish red, rounded glands about one-fourth of an inch in diameter. They are located behind each side of the thyroid, two near the top of the lobes and two near the bottom.

The hormones secreted by the thyroid are rich in iodine, a trace mineral usually found in salt from the sea. One of these hormones, thyroxin, is extremely important. If the thyroid secretes too much of it, the body's organs work at an accelerated pace, much like a motor given too much gas, resulting in a condition known as hyperthyroidism. Its symptoms are extreme nervousness, weight loss, rapid pulse, and bulging eyes. Eventually, heart failure results from the overworking of the body's systems in their attempt to handle all the speeded up organic functions. If too little thyroxin is secreted, often due to a lack of iodine in the diet, a condition called hypothyroidism exists. People suffering from this may exhibit such symptoms as goiter, which is an enlarged thyroid gland, physical and mental sluggishness, decreased body temperature, and puffiness in the face and hands.

The parathyroid glands produce the hormones that control the calcium and phosphorus levels in the body, especially important in muscle control and teeth and bone formation. If the parathyroid glands are underactive, the blood-calcium level falls and the phosphorus level rises. This produces two major problems: tetany, a condition of spontaneous and uncontrollable muscle spasms in the wrists and ankles; and bone calcium loss, due to the parathyroids signaling the bones to release their calcium into the blood in order to raise the blood-calcium levels. This release of bone calcium is one of the causes of osteoporosis, or brittle bones, in women after they have reached menopause. When the body no longer produces the estrogen that regulates hormone flow, the parathyroid glands slow or stop secreting their important hormones; therefore, the bones are triggered to release their calcium and they become weak and brittle. The body is so sensitive to and dependent on these tiny glands that, if they are injured or removed surgically, tetany often sets in within twenty-four hours.

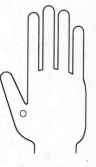

BOTH HANDS

A workout of the thyroid and parathyroid glands through reflexology is primarily a regulatory function. It can help keep the glands active and working at their proper pace, which is vital to the overall tranquility of the body. There are reflex areas on both palms and both soles. Since the parathyroid glands are just behind the thyroid-gland lobes, their reflex areas fall in much the same place and they are stimulated when the thyroid reflex is worked. On the palms, the reflexes are on the inner edge of the base of the thumbs. On the soles, the reflexes are on the lower edge of the pad at the base of the big toes, down from the crease between the big and second toes.

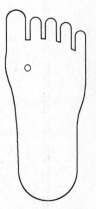

BOTH FEET

TECHNIQUES

Since both the thyroid and parathyroid glands are located along the body's midline, with lobes on each side of the neck, their reflex points can be found on both palms and both soles. Rather than concentrating on only one side, be sure to work on both the right and left sides. Use a firm, rolling pressure as you slowly work the reflexes, but do not cause any real discomfort as you do so. Carefully note any tenderness or soreness in the reflexes, as these may indicate some form of distress in the thyroid or parathyroid glands that might interfere with their regulatory tasks. Visualize these glands and their various functions while you are working on their reflexes. Breathe rhythmically, inhaling as you press the reflex and exhaling as you release the pressure.

THE HANDS — The reflex points for the thyroid and parathyroid glands are on the palms, located on the inner edge of the base of the thumbs, near the crease between the thumbs and the index fingers, about three-fourths of the way to the wrists. Be careful not to bruise the tissues as you use your thumb in a firm, rolling press against the points. Start with a light pressure, release it slightly, then increase it as you begin the next press. You are going to do this seven times on each palm. Increase the pressure each time, letting up a little between presses. Do not stop the pressure altogether until you have finished the thyroid and parathyroid workout.

THE FEET — The thyroid and parathyroid glands have their reflex points on the soles of both feet. These are found at the lower, inside edge the pad at the base of the big toes, almost straight down from the crease between the big and second toes. This is a very sensitive spot, so be careful not to bruise any tissues, or you might find yourself limping after a workout. Using a technique identical to that for the hands, you are going to work the reflexes on each sole seven times. Use your thumb in a pressing, rolling motion, starting with only a little pressure and gradually increasing it as you go. Release the pressure a bit between presses, but do not let up completely until the thyroid and parathyroid workout is finished.

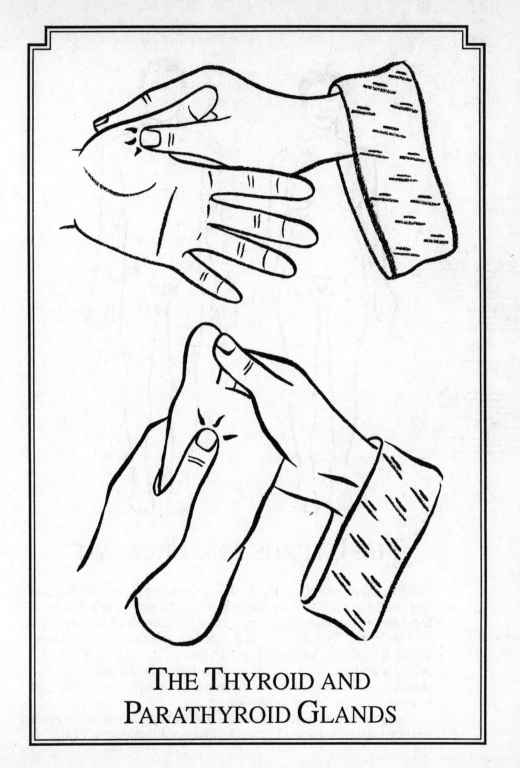

THE THYROID AND
PARATHYROID GLANDS

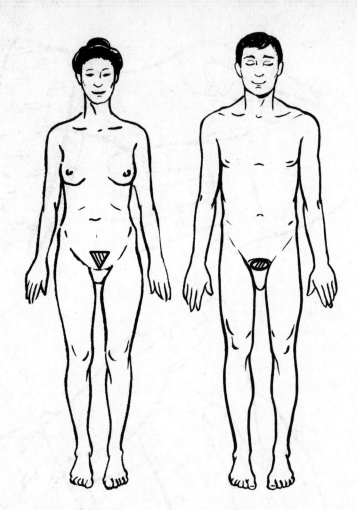

THE UTERUS AND PROSTATE

The uterus, or womb, is the female organ that receives a mature egg from an ovary. When the egg enters the uterus, if it has been fertilized, it is housed and nurtured by the uterus until it develops into an infant. The prostate is the male equivalent of the uterus. While it does not house sperm, it secretes an alkaline fluid that protects and nurtures sperm so that, after ejaculation, they can survive while they travel up the vagina, through the uterus, and into the fallopian tubes to fertilize an egg.

The prostate is partly muscular and partly glandular. In most healthy men it is shaped like a chestnut but a little larger in size. It can swell when infections are present; however, and in men over the age of fifty, the prostate often becomes enlarged and sometimes cancerous. The reasons for this are still not known, although hormonal changes due to aging are suspected.

The uterus, a fist-sized sac shaped like a tilted, upside-down pear, is mostly thick muscle. It has two parts — a neck, or cervix, and a body. The cervix is a tight, hollow cylinder through which menstrual discharges flow, sperm enter the uterus, and an infant is born. The area inside the rounded body of the uterus is actually quite small and is shaped like an upside-down triangle. The two top vertices lead off to the fallopian tubes, through which a mature egg travels from the ovary, while the lower vertex ends at the cervix. A mucous membrane lines this triangle and is designed to hold a fertilized egg. If the egg that arrives is infertile, the uterus receives a signal to discharge the lining and the egg, resulting in the periodic flow of blood known as menstruation. If the egg is fertile, the lining thickens and the egg develops into a fetus. As the fetus grows in size the uterus stretches. When the fetus is fully developed, the uterus undergoes a series of contractions that force the infant down through the cervix and vagina and out into the world.

The prostate is located in males at the bottom of the bladder. It partially encircles the urethra, the tube through which urine flows out of the body. When the prostate becomes enlarged, it can interfere with or even cut off this flow of urine, causing great discomfort and endangering the general health of the body. Therapy with female hormones and surgery are often the solutions to an enlarged prostate. Until recently, prostate surgical techniques damaged nerves, resulting in impotence, but advances in microsurgery can now circumvent this problem in most cases.

The uterus, located between the bladder and the rectum, is susceptible to problems such as infections, polyps, cysts, fibroid tumors, cancers, and a condition known as prolapse, where the supporting abdominal muscles are too weak, causing the entire uterus to "fall" and the cervix to protrude from the vagina. Many of these conditions can be treated, and pap smears are helpful in detecting some of the cancers.

A workout of the uterus or prostate reflexes can help keep these body parts in peak condition so that they can perform their reproductive functions and resist disease. The reflexes for the uterus in women and the prostate in men are in the same place, on the sides of both feet and both wrists. On the feet the points are in the pockets under the inner ankle bones, while on the wrists they can be found in the small indentations on the edge under the thumbs, just below the base of the palms.

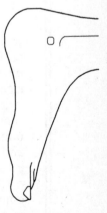

BOTH HANDS

BOTH FEET

TECHNIQUES

The reflex points for the uterus and the prostate are in the same places on the hands and feet. The points on a female are for the uterus, while those on males are for the prostate. Concentrating on the points will produce the most direct results, but, since these are only parts of the reproductive system, it is a good idea to work out the reflexes of related organs as well. Use care and be very gentle the first few times you work the points, especially when there is a pregnancy. Visualize the uterus or prostate, and inhale as you press the reflex, exhaling as you release the pressure. When working out the points, note any tenderness — this may alert you to some form of distress. Be careful not to cause any real pain when applying pressure.

THE HANDS — Since the uterus and the prostate are located in the middle of the body, there are reflex points on both hands. Do not work on just one hand in a workout session — do both. The reflex is at the base of the palm, actually on the wrist, in the little hollow formed between the bone at the base of the palm, straight down from the index finger and the bone at the bottom of the arm. Encircle the wrist so that your index finger is on the reflex. Press gently but firmly with your index finger, then release the pressure slightly. On the next press, exert a little more pressure, then pull back again. You are going to do this seven times to each reflex point. Gradually increase your pressure, with slight releases between presses. Be sure not to let up on the pressure completely until you have finished the workout.

THE FEET — The uterus and prostate reflex points on both feet are in the hollows under the inner ankle bones, just above the middle of each hollow. These are extremely sensitive areas, so be careful when working on them, and be sure to work both the right and the left foot in a session. Using a technique identical to that for the hands, you are going to stimulate these points seven times. Place your thumb on the hollow under the inside ankle bone and press firmly on the reflex. The first time, press slowly and gently. Release the pressure slightly, then begin your next press. Increase the pressure on the subsequent presses, backing off a little between them, but do not let up on the pressure completely until the end of the uterus and prostate workout.

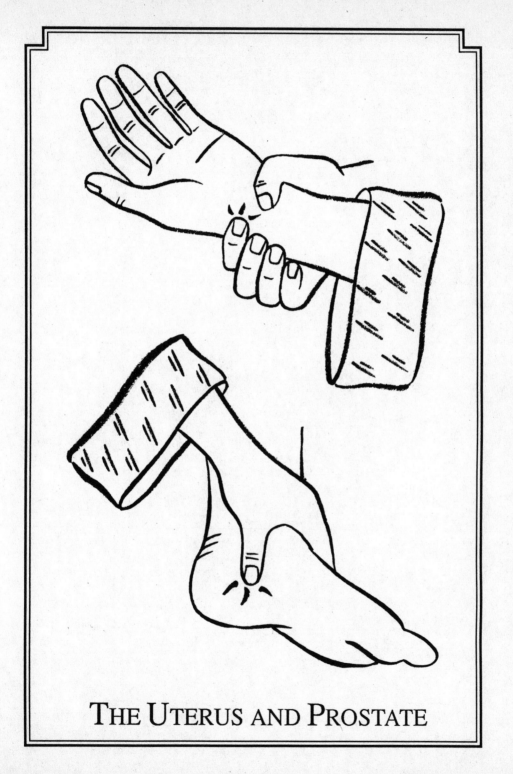

THE UTERUS AND PROSTATE

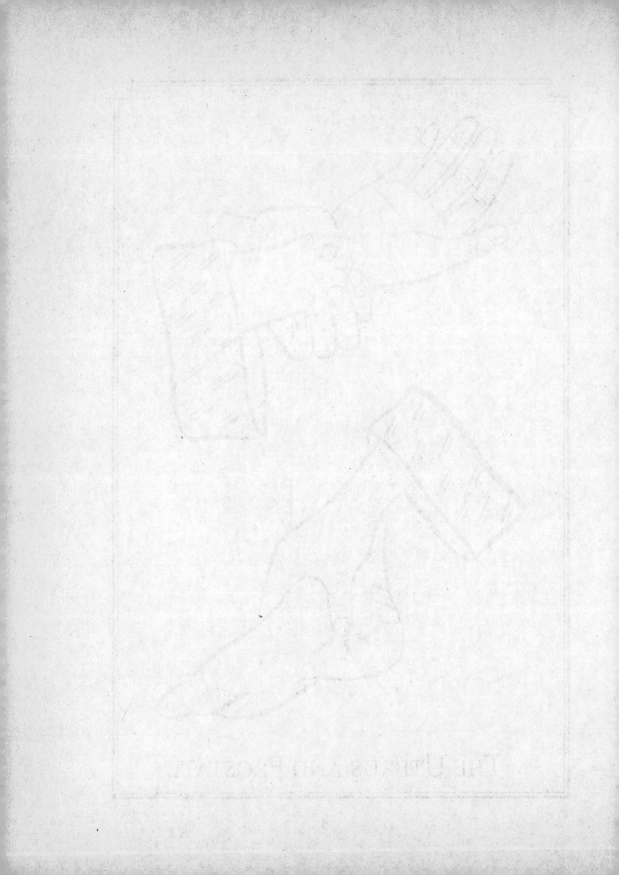

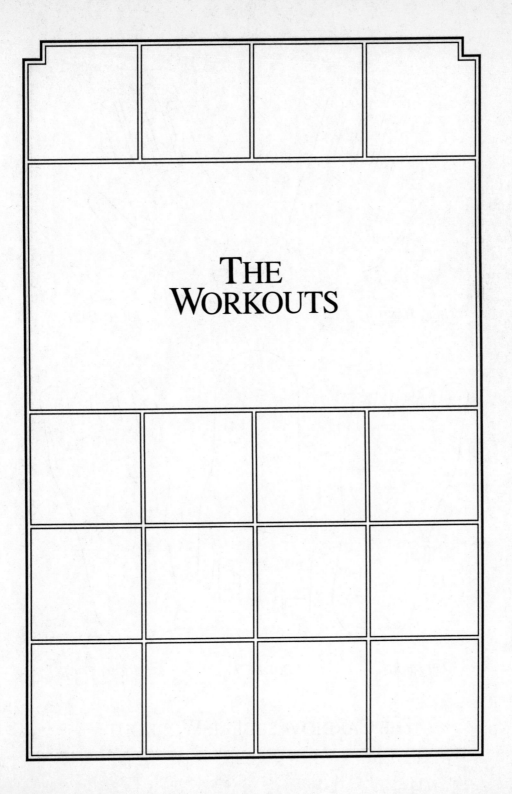

THE
WORKOUTS

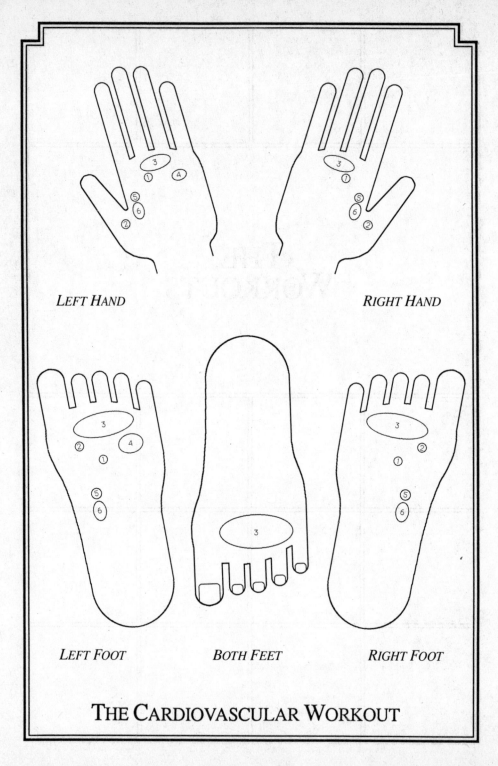

LEFT HAND

RIGHT HAND

LEFT FOOT

BOTH FEET

RIGHT FOOT

THE CARDIOVASCULAR WORKOUT

THE CARDIOVASCULAR WORKOUT

SEVEN MINUTES — THREE TIMES A WEEK

The cardiovascular system, the system made up of the heart, lungs, and blood vessels, is directly responsible for the health and nutrition of the body. The cells of the brain, muscles, organs, bones, and skin all receive oxygen and nutrients from the blood pumped through and around them by the heart. The blood also transports toxic wastes from these cells to the appropriate organs for disposal.

A strong and healthy cardiovascular system affects the quality of life and the lifespan itself. Diseases of the cardiovascular system are among the major causes of death and disability in the United States. Diet and exercise play the primary role in keeping blood vessels clear of blockage, the circulation at its most efficient, and the heart — the body's strongest and most important muscle — in peak condition.

The Cardiovascular Workout is an excellent adjunct to your normal exercise program. Alternate it with the Tone-up Workout just before you exercise, to improve your stamina. Begin with the left hand or foot, working the first reflex area listed below, then move over to the same reflex area on the right hand and foot. Alternate sides as you work the reflexes in the order listed. Remember, visualize the parts of the body you are stimulating, and coordinate the pressure with your breathing patterns.

1. The Solar Plexus and Diaphragm Reflexes (seven times each, left and right sides) stimulate these parts to induce a strong breathing pattern.
2. The Thyroid and Parathyroid Gland Reflexes (seven times each, left and right sides) stimulate these glands to regulate the body's metabolic rate and pulse rate while controlling muscle tension.
3. The Lung Reflexes (seven times each, left and right sides) stimulate the lungs to exchange toxic carbon dioxide in the blood for the oxygen necessary for efficient metabolic reactions.
4. The Heart Reflex (seven times, left side only) stimulates the heart, regulating the cardiovascular action that pumps blood throughout the body.
5. The Adrenal Gland Reflexes (seven times each, left and right sides) prompt the adrenals to secrete hormones that enhance the muscle tone of the heart and regulate blood pressure by controlling sodium and potassium levels.
6. The Kidney Reflexes (seven times each, left and right sides) encourage the kidneys to process wastes out of the blood while regulating fluid balances that affect blood pressure.
1. The Solar Plexus and Diaphragm Reflexes (seven times each, left and right sides) signal these mid-body parts to stabilize proper breathing action.

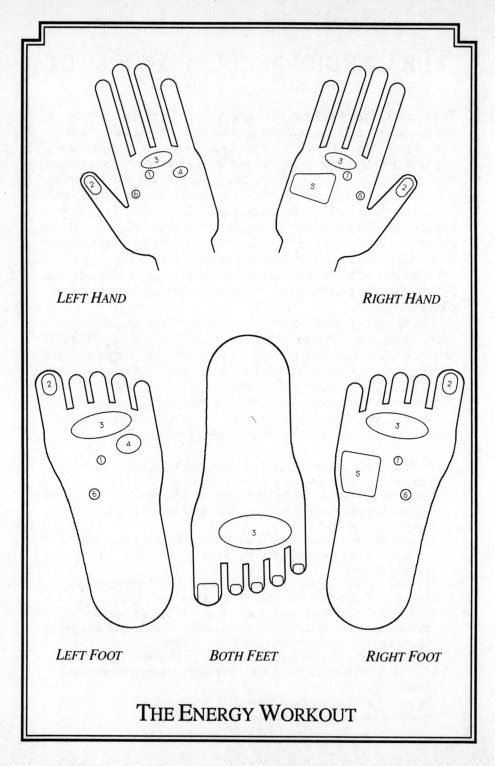

LEFT HAND   RIGHT HAND

LEFT FOOT   BOTH FEET   RIGHT FOOT

THE ENERGY WORKOUT

THE ENERGY WORKOUT

SEVEN MINUTES — MORNINGS OR WHENEVER FATIGUED

When the body and mind are alert, the emotional atmosphere is one of enthusiasm and the mental processes become clear. These are useful qualities in daily life and important professional characteristics. People who are alert enough to seize opportunities or sense problems, responding quickly and constructively, are those most frequently rewarded.

A little zing of energy can make all the difference in the routine tasks of the day. Energetic people tend to be concerned, quick-witted, and capable of decisive action. Furthermore, vigorous and industrious people seem to have an easier time focusing their interest on others, rather than on themselves. This strengthens the social networks that support personal and career development. They are also better able to express their feelings openly, reducing the stress in their lives.

The Energy Workout is a simple exercise that can be performed at the start of the day or whenever a burst of energy is needed. Work the reflex areas in the order that they are listed. Begin with the first reflex area on the left hand or foot, then move over to the same reflex area on the right side. Both the hands and the feet will yield the same results, but try to work the feet in the morning, before you get out of bed. Remember, coordinate the pressure with your breathing, and visualize the parts of the body that you are stimulating.

1. The Solar Plexus and Diaphragm Reflexes (seven times each, left and right sides) trigger the solar plexus to relax the body and set up a strong breathing pattern.
2. The Brain Reflexes (seven times each, left and right sides) prompt the brain to enhance its neurological functions.
3. The Lung Reflexes (seven times each, left and right sides) invigorate the body by stimulating the lungs to increase the oxygen level in the blood.
4. The Heart Reflex (seven times, left side only) stimulates the heart as it pumps oxygen-rich blood from the lungs to the brain.
5. The Liver Reflex (seven times, right side only) stimulates the liver to release stored energy nutrients into the bloodstream.
6. The Adrenal Gland Reflexes (seven times each, left and right sides) induce these glands to release epinephrine (Adrenalin) to eliminate fatigue and speed up reaction time.
1. The Solar Plexus and Diaphragm Reflexes (seven times each, left and right sides) prompt the solar plexus to send nervous signals that encourage a feeling of calmness and clarity.

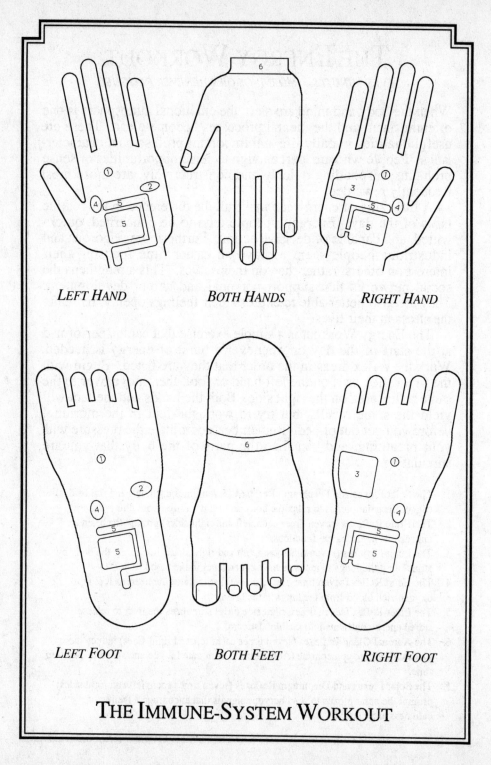

LEFT HAND   BOTH HANDS   RIGHT HAND

LEFT FOOT   BOTH FEET   RIGHT FOOT

THE IMMUNE-SYSTEM WORKOUT

THE IMMUNE-SYSTEM WORKOUT

SEVEN MINUTES — TWO TIMES A WEEK
OR WHEN DEVELOPING AN ILLNESS

Immunity, the body's ability to resist infection, can be inherited genetically or acquired through exposure or inoculation. When the body develops an infection, it triggers the formation of antibodies, the substances that fight germs and their effects. Immunity to a disease exists when the body's defense systems contain antibodies to that disease, but immunity can be adversely affected when the body's physical condition is poor. Inadequate diet, stress, and exhaustion all deplete the body's resources and weaken the immune system. At times, antibodies to certain germs, particularly viruses, do not develop at all. In some serious illnesses, certain microorganisms seem to neutralize the body's immune system. Acquired Immune Deficiency Syndrome, better known as AIDS, is one example of this type of systemic failure.

The Immune-System Workout is designed to stimulate the parts of the body that are most responsible for fighting disease. Try it when you feel a cold or flu coming on: It might not stop the illness, but it will probably decrease its duration and severity. Stimulate the reflex areas in the order listed below, visualizing the parts you are stimulating and coordinating the pressure with your breathing. Start with the first reflex area on the left hand or foot, then move over to the same reflex on the right side.

1. The Solar Plexus and Diaphragm Reflexes (seven times each, left and right sides) stimulate the solar plexus to strengthen abdominal responses and set up a good breathing pattern.
2. The Spleen Reflex (seven times, left side only) stimulates the spleen to perform its specific immunological functions, while recycling red blood cells.
3. The Liver Reflex (seven times, right side only) prompts the liver to filter wastes and produce antibodies, tasks vital to the body's defense system.
4. The Kidney Reflexes (seven times each, left and right sides) speed the purification of the blood by prompting the kidneys to process toxic wastes.
5. The Intestine Reflexes (seven times each, left and right sides) spur the intestines to dispose of toxins and wastes from the body.
6. The Lymphatic System Reflexes (seven times each, left and right sides) mobilize the lymph nodes to release disease-fighting cells throughout the body to provide a vital line of defense against infection.
1. The Solar Plexus and Diaphragm Reflexes (seven times each, left and right sides) trigger the solar plexus to send signals that relax abdominal muscles and organs, fighting stress that weakens the immune system.

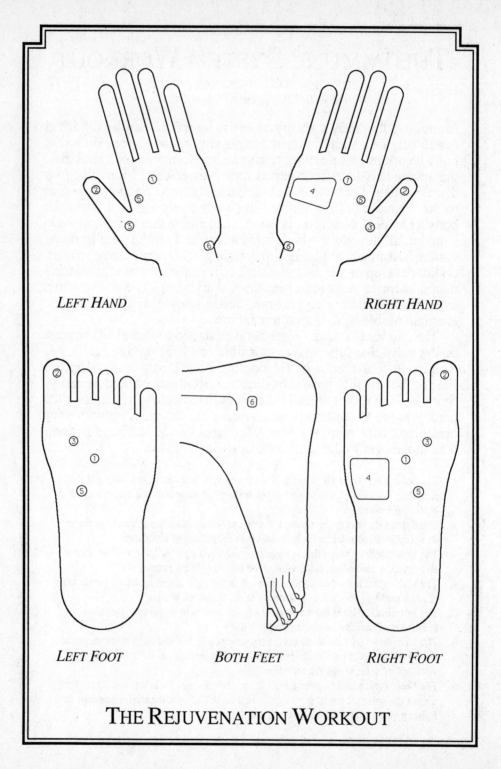

LEFT HAND

RIGHT HAND

LEFT FOOT

BOTH FEET

RIGHT FOOT

THE REJUVENATION WORKOUT

THE REJUVENATION WORKOUT

SEVEN MINUTES — TWO TIMES A WEEK

The cells of the body are continuously replaced by new ones as we age. In fact, during a lifetime we will shed and regrow the outer layers of our skin nearly one thousand times. Over a seven-year period, the body completely replaces itself, with the exception of nerve cells, which do not regenerate at all. The process of regeneration is still a mystery locked in the DNA, but we do know that hormones play a critical role in the process.

Hormones are chemical messengers secreted by glands and sent to other parts of the body to regulate their functions. Hormones control the growth and development of the body from the fetal stage through old age; the reproductive processes; and, most important, the body's ability to resist infection and disease. Therefore, keeping the glands that secrete hormones in peak condition is the key to good health and youthful vigor at all ages.

The Rejuvenation Workout stimulates the primary hormone-producing glands, encouraging them to be alert and responsive to the body's needs. Work the reflex areas listed below in the order that they are presented. Start by working the first reflex area on the left hand or foot, then go over to the same area on the right hand or foot. Remember, coordinate the pressure with your breathing, and visualize the glands you are stimulating.

1. The Solar Plexus and Diaphragm Reflexes (seven times each, left and right sides) prompt the solar plexus to send signals that regulate breathing and relax the body.
2. The Pituitary Gland Reflexes (seven times each, left and right sides) stimulate the pituitary to secrete hormones that align the functions of all the other glands in the body.
3. The Thyroid and Parathyroid Gland Reflexes (seven times each, left and right sides) stimulate these glands to produce hormones that regulate metabolic rates, enhance muscle tone, and encourage teeth and bone formation.
4. The Liver Reflex (seven times, right side only) stimulates the liver to process nutrients, remove wastes, and produce antibodies to enhance the immune system.
5. The Adrenal Gland Reflexes (seven times each, left and right sides) prompt the adrenals to align the body's water and mineral balance and to secrete epinephrine (Adrenalin) for alertness and quick energy.
6. The Ovary and Testicle Reflexes (seven times each, left and right sides) stimulate these gonads to produce hormones that control reproductive cycles and enhance youthful vitality.
1. The Solar Plexus and Diaphragm Reflexes (seven times each, left and right sides) trigger the solar plexus to send signals that soothe anxiety, depression, and other effects of stress.

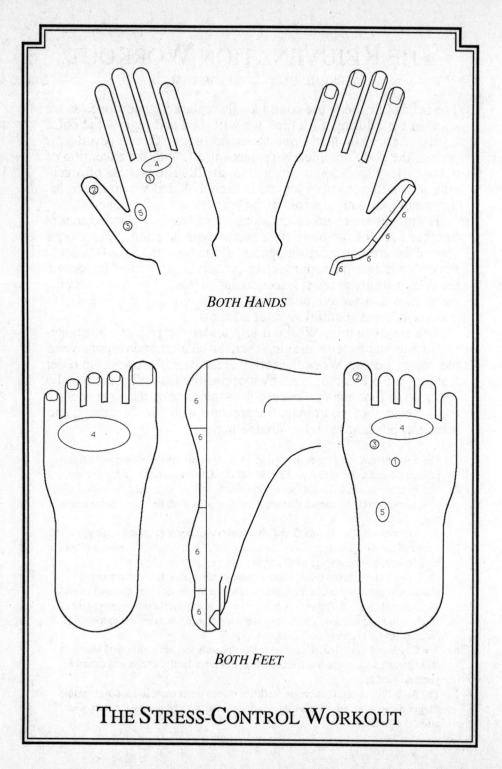

BOTH HANDS

BOTH FEET

THE STRESS-CONTROL WORKOUT

THE STRESS-CONTROL WORKOUT

SEVEN MINUTES — EVENINGS OR WHENEVER TENSE

Stress, one of the least understood conditions in modern life, permeates almost every human activity. Professions involving financial or personal risk-taking, or the constant pressure of deadlines, are extremely stressful. Personal relationships that are in emotional transition also cause intense stress, particularly when feelings must be concealed.

While some stress is beneficial to survival, constant stress is extremely debilitating and can lead to sleepless nights, poor digestion, and feelings of tension and irritability. Recent studies show a direct correlation between levels of stress and heart disease, peptic ulcers, migraine headaches, suicide, and high blood pressure. Nevertheless, stress control is surprisingly easy to achieve and can produce remarkable changes in your personal, physical, and emotional well-being.

The Stress-Control Workout should be performed whenever you feel tense. Work the reflex areas in the order that they are listed, starting with the first reflex area on the left hand or foot, then going to the same reflex area on the right side. One of the best ways to do this particular workout is to have a friend help you. Do not forget to coordinate the pressure with your breathing and visualize the parts of the body that you are stimulating.

1. The Solar Plexus and Diaphragm Reflexes (seven times each, left and right sides) prompt these parts to set up a regular breathing pattern and channel relaxing signals to the muscles and organs in the abdomen.
2. The Pituitary Gland Reflexes (seven times each, left and right sides) stimulate the pituitary to align specific hormonal balances in the body, bringing about a calming sensation.
3. The Thyroid and Parathyroid Gland Reflexes (seven times each, left and right sides) encourage these glands to bring muscle tension into balance, which affects the overall tranquility of the body.
4. The Lung Reflexes (seven times each, left and right sides) prompt the lungs to increase the blood's oxygen level, thus enhancing metabolic processes that refresh and nurture the body.
5. The Kidney Reflexes (seven times each, left and right sides) trigger the kidneys to align the fluid balances that affect blood pressure.
6. The Spine Reflexes (seven times each, left and right sides) prompt the spinal cord, with about half the body's nerve cells, to soothe nervous responses.
1. The Solar Plexus and Diaphragm Reflexes (seven times each, left and right sides) induce the solar plexus to send signals that leave the body feeling pleasantly relaxed.

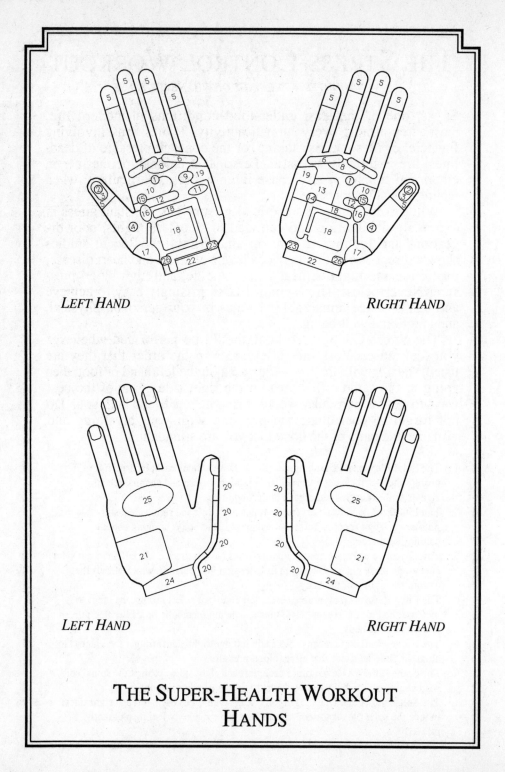

LEFT HAND

RIGHT HAND

LEFT HAND

RIGHT HAND

THE SUPER-HEALTH WORKOUT
HANDS

THE SUPER-HEALTH WORKOUT

THIRTY MINUTES — TWO TIMES A WEEK
(UP TO FORTY-FIVE MINUTES IF USING A TROUBLESHOOTING APPLICATION)

As a machine, the body is very peculiar — it actually wears out faster the less it is used. Although it is true that the aging process contributes to the degeneration of the body over time, recent studies indicate that physical efficiency can actually be increased throughout life with a good diet and physical conditioning. These same two factors appear to directly contribute to longer life spans and, combined with a flexible attitude and adaptable lifestyle, they even increase the levels of intellectual performance.

Physical condition is not limited to just the muscles and the cardiovascular system — it includes the organs, the skin, the glands, the bones, and every other part of the body. While a regular program of physical exercise keeps muscles toned and the cardiovascular system tuned, the organs are seldom stimulated to their capacity. A physical workout contributes in part to their health, but a reflexology workout can affect them directly.

The Super-Health Workout takes more time than the others, but it is a complete reflexology session, similar to that given by a physical therapist. To perform the workout, stimulate the reflexes in the order listed on the next page. Start with the first reflex area listed and work the left hand or foot, then move to the same reflex area on the right side. Remember, coordinate the pressure with your breathing, and visualize each body part as you are stimulating it. If you have a specific body part you would like to work on, increase the number of times you stimulate that reflex from seven to fourteen when you come to it in the Super-Health Workout.

If you are trying to clear up or prevent specific physical disorders that are listed in Part Three, "Troubleshooting," this is the workout to use. Look up the disorder and its reflexology formula. Then perform the Super-Health Workout as usual; but whenever you come to a reflex that is in your Troubleshooting formula, increase the number of times you press that reflex from seven to fourteen. You will find that performing the Super-Health/Troubleshooting Workout twice a week is probably ample to help prevent disorders that concern you. If you are fighting a specific health problem, then you may want to increase the workout frequency to once a day until the condition subsides.

LEFT FOOT

RIGHT FOOT

BOTH FEET

THE SUPER-HEALTH WORKOUT
FEET

THE SUPER-HEALTH WORKOUT

1. The Solar Plexus and Diaphragm Reflexes (seven times each, left and right sides).
2. The Pituitary Gland Reflexes (seven times each, left and right sides).
3. The Brain Reflexes (seven times each, left and right sides).
4. The Thyroid and Parathyroid Gland Reflexes (seven times each, left and right sides).
5. The Sinus Reflexes (seven times each, left and right sides).
6. The Ear Reflexes (seven times each, left and right sides).
7. The Eye Reflexes (seven times each, left and right sides).
8. The Lung Reflexes (seven times each, left and right sides).
9. The Heart Reflex (seven times, left side only).
10. The Stomach Reflexes (seven times each, left and right sides).
11. The Spleen Reflex (seven times, left side only).
12. The Pancreas Reflexes (seven times each, left and right sides).
13. The Liver Reflex (seven times, right side only).
14. The Gallbladder Reflex (seven times, right side only).
15. The Adrenal Gland Reflexes (seven times each, left and right sides).
16. The Kidney Reflexes (seven times each, left and right sides).
17. The Bladder, Ureter, and Urethra Reflexes (seven times each, left and right sides).
18. The Intestine Reflexes (seven times each, left and right sides).
19. The Arm and Shoulder Reflexes (seven times each, left and right sides).
20. The Spine Reflexes (seven times each, left and right sides).
21. The Hip, Thigh, and Leg Reflexes (seven times each, left and right sides).
22. The Sciatic Nerve Reflexes (seven times each, left and right sides).
23. The Ovary and Testicle Reflexes (seven times each, left and right sides).
24. The Lymphatic System Reflexes (seven times each, left and right sides).
25. The Breast Reflexes (seven times each, left and right sides).
26. The Uterus and Prostate Reflexes (seven times each, left and right sides).
1. The Solar Plexus and Diaphragm Reflexes (seven times each, left and right sides).

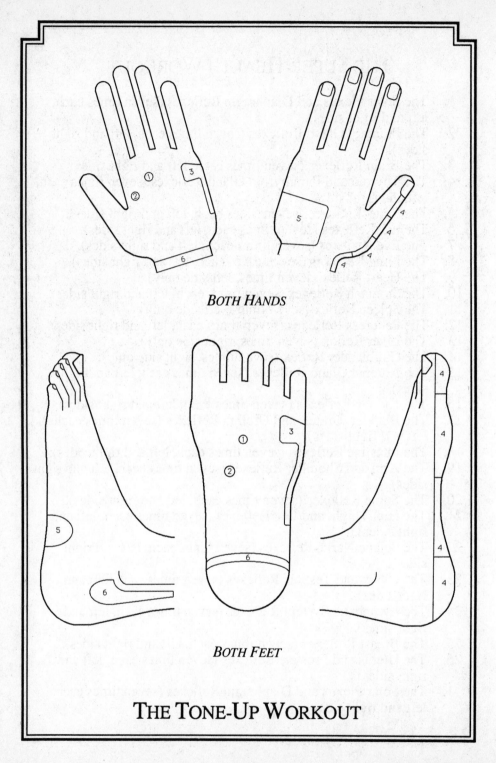

BOTH HANDS

BOTH FEET

THE TONE-UP WORKOUT

THE TONE-UP WORKOUT

SEVEN MINUTES — THREE TIMES A WEEK

Every facet of life, from mental health to longevity, is affected by physical fitness. People who are not fit are fatigued more often, are not as mentally efficient, and succumb more frequently to colds and flu for longer lengths of time than those who stay in shape. This is particularly true for people in sedentary jobs who believe they are too tired or too busy to exercise.

The physical benefits of exercise are readily apparent in good muscle tone, a trim figure, increased stamina, and improved coordination. Furthermore, exercise creates feelings of well-being that make work more efficient and less stressful. Generally, life feels better in a well-toned body — one that is healthy, alert, and comfortable to wear.

The Tone-up Workout stimulates the skeletal structure, the muscles, and nervous system, as well as the major joints in the body. Try alternating it with the Cardiovascular Workout before your physical-exercise program. Begin with the first reflex area listed below, working on your left hand or foot. Then move to the same reflex area on your right hand or foot. Continue alternating the reflexes on the left and right as you work them in the order listed below. Be sure to coordinate the pressure with your breathing and visualize the body parts you are stimulating.

1. The Solar Plexus and Diaphragm Reflexes (seven times each, left and right sides) trigger these parts to set up a strong breathing pattern and stimulate all the nerves in the abdominal area.
2. The Adrenal Gland Reflexes (seven times each, left and right sides) stimulate the adrenals to secrete hormones that are essential to the metabolic functions in the muscles and nerves.
3. The Arm and Shoulder Reflexes (seven times each, left and right sides) stimulate the muscles and nerves of the upper limbs, and increase blood circulation in the arms, the shoulders, the elbows, and the wrists.
4. The Spine Reflexes (seven times each, left and right sides) prompt the spine and spinal cord to align nervous responses and enhance spinal flexibility.
5. The Hip, Thigh, and Leg Reflexes (seven times each, left and right sides) stimulate the muscles and nerves of the lower limbs and increase blood circulation in the thighs, legs, hips, knees, and ankles.
6. The Sciatic Nerve Reflexes (seven times each, left and right sides) trigger the sciatic nerves to stimulate the muscles and nerves used in standing, walking, and balancing.
1. The Solar Plexus and Diaphragm Reflexes (seven times each, left and right sides) prompt this nerve bundle to put the body into an aware, coordinated state.

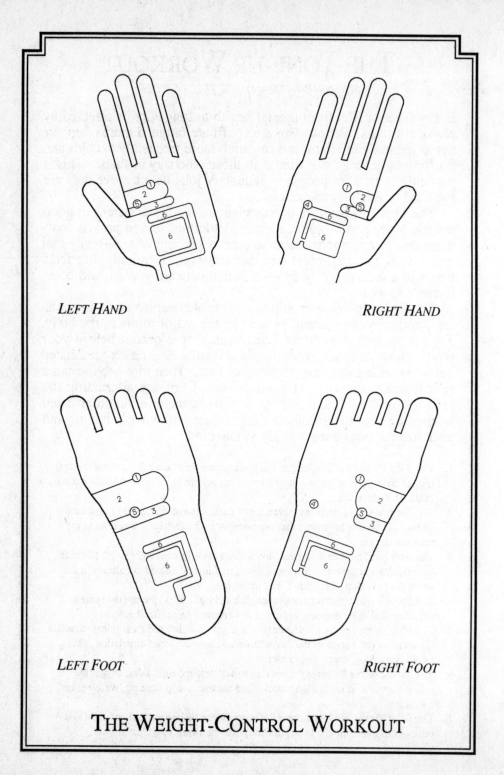

LEFT HAND   RIGHT HAND

LEFT FOOT   RIGHT FOOT

THE WEIGHT-CONTROL WORKOUT

THE WEIGHT-CONTROL WORKOUT

SEVEN MINUTES — DAILY

It is estimated that over half the people in the United States are overweight. Significant weight gain tends to take place at particular times in life: Men tend to gain excess weight between the ages of twenty-five and forty, with a significant increase over the age of forty; women tend to gain weight after their twenties, during pregnancy, and during menopause. Yet the most common reason for a gain in weight is eating too many calories and then not getting enough exercise to burn them off. These excess calories are then stored in the body as fat. Statistics indicate that the risks of death and disease, particularly cardiovascular diseases and certain cancers, increase along with an increase in weight.

The Weight-Control Workout stimulates the organs of the digestive system that help regulate nutritional intake and speed the eliminatory processes. Start with the first reflex area listed below on the left hand or foot, then move over to the same area on the right side. The reflexes on both the hands and the feet will give the same results, but try to work the reflexes on the feet at least once a week. Coordinate the pressure with your breathing and visualize the parts of the body you are stimulating.

1. The Solar Plexus and Diaphragm Reflexes (seven times each, left and right sides) trigger the solar plexus and diaphragm to initiate efficient breathing and send metabolic information to all the organs in the abdomen.
2. The Stomach Reflexes (seven times each, left and right sides) stimulate the stomach's food-mashing action and speed the release of important digestive juices.
3. The Pancreas Reflexes (seven times each, left and right sides) induce the pancreas to secrete juices that quickly break down carbohydrates while balancing the blood-sugar level.
4. The Gallbladder Reflex (seven times, right side only) stimulates the gallbladder to release the bile that emulsifies fats and acts as a mild laxative to speed waste elimination.
5. The Adrenal Gland Reflexes (seven times each, left and right sides) prompt the adrenals to release hormones that regulate metabolic functions and enhance the muscle tone of the intestines for rapid elimination.
6. The Intestine Reflexes (seven times each, left and right sides) stimulate and enhance the actions of the intestines, the primary organs of waste elimination.
1. The Solar Plexus and Diaphragm Reflexes (seven times each, left and right sides) prompt the solar plexus to send nervous signals that reinforce feelings of calm and well-being.

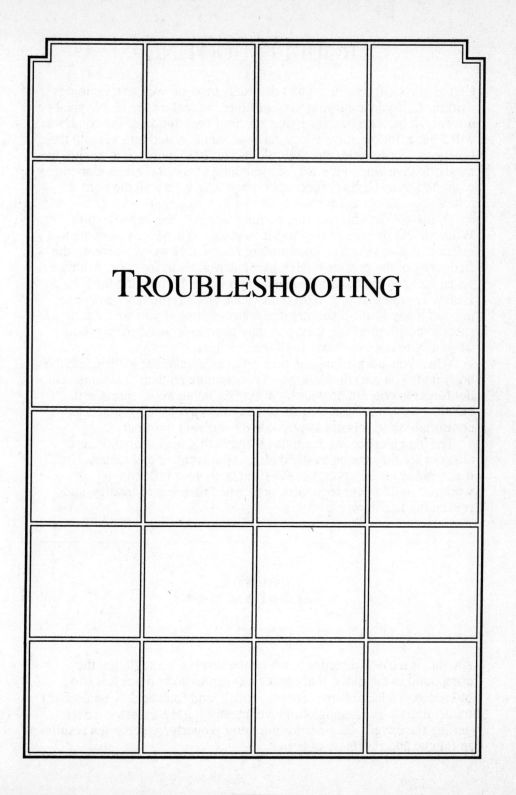

TROUBLESHOOTING

TROUBLESHOOTING

Certain physical conditions and disorders respond well to reflexology workouts. If you are trying to clear up or prevent a specific physical disorder, look it up in this section. A brief description of the condition will appear, followed by a formula — a list of related reflexes and their functions. Since reflexology employs a holistic approach to health, the most effective way to use a Troubleshooting formula is in conjunction with the Super-Health Workout on page 130, where all the body's reflexology points are engaged.

To use the Troubleshooting formulas, turn to the Super-Health Workout and prepare to perform it as usual. Whenever you come to a reflex that is in your Troubleshooting formula, however, increase the frequency of the presses on that particular reflex to fourteen, from the seven indicated in the Super-Health Workout. Performing the Super-Health/Troubleshooting Workout twice a week is probably ample to prevent many of the disorders that concern you. If you are fighting a specific health problem, then you may want to increase the workout frequency to once each day until the condition clears up.

When you are working on your reflexes, remember to visualize the body parts you are stimulating and concentrate on their functions. Do not forget to coordinate your breathing, inhaling as you press and exhaling as you release the pressure, and always make yourself as comfortable and relaxed as possible during your workout.

The Troubleshooting formulas listed in this section are not cure-alls; nor are they meant to stand alone as preventive techniques. Use them, rather, as adjuncts, not substitutes, to your reflexology workouts and to your regular or prescribed methods of treating and preventing health problems.

ACNE
(*see* SKIN DISORDERS)

ANEMIA

Anemia is a blood disorder in which the level of hemoglobin, the compound in the blood that carries oxygen to body tissues, is low, often due to a lack of iron, copper, cobalt, and folic acid (vitamin B12) in the diet. A low hemoglobin level means that the tissues are not getting the oxygen they need to function properly, which often results in fatigue and shortness of breath.

1. The Spleen Reflex (fourteen times, left side only) stimulates the spleen, which acts as a storehouse for iron, to recycle hemoglobin from damaged or dead red blood cells.
2. The Liver Reflex (fourteen times, right side only) stimulates the liver to store and release copper, iron, and vitamin B12 as they are needed.

ARTHRITIS

This inflammation of one or more joints in the body is due to a variety of factors that include aging, obesity, and stress-related tension.

1. The Solar Plexus and Diaphragm Reflexes (fourteen times each, left and right sides) prompt these body parts to fight stress by signaling the nerves of the body to relax.
2. The Thyroid and Parathyroid Gland Reflexes (fourteen times each, left and right sides) stimulate these glands to secrete hormones that regulate muscle tension.
3. The Adrenal Gland Reflexes (fourteen times each, left and right sides) induce these glands to secrete hydrocortisone, the natural form of cortisone that reduces tissue inflammation.
4. The Kidney Reflexes (fourteen times each, left and right sides) trigger the kidneys to process fluid wastes that collect around the joints.
5. The Arm and Shoulder Reflexes (fourteen times each, left and right sides) stimulate the shoulder, elbow, wrist, and other joints, increasing their blood circulation and toning-up the muscles and nerves around them.
6. The Spine Reflexes (fourteen times each, left and right sides) prompt the spine to enhance its flexibility and the spinal cord to regulate its nervous responses.
7. The Hip, Thigh, and Leg Reflexes (fourteen times each, left and right sides) stimulate the joints and the lower limbs, increasing their blood circulation and toning-up the surrounding muscles and nerves.

ASTHMA

This condition is one of severe difficulty in breathing due to allergies, emotional stress, and a number of other factors.

1. The Solar Plexus and Diaphragm Reflexes (fourteen times each, left and right sides) trigger the solar plexus and diaphragm to regulate breathing and to signal the body to relax and overcome panic reactions and feelings of anxiety.
2. The Pituitary Gland Reflexes (fourteen times each, left and right

sides) stimulate the gland to secrete the hormones that control the functions of all the other glands in the body.
3. The Lung Reflexes (fourteen times each, left and right sides) encourage the lungs and bronchial tubes to function normally, without constriction.
4. The Adrenal Gland Reflexes (fourteen times each, left and right sides) trigger the adrenals to secrete epinephrine (Adrenalin), which opens up the air passages, and hydrocortisone, a natural form of cortisone, which reduces tissue inflammation.
5. The Intestine Reflexes (fourteen times each, left and right sides) stimulate the small and large intestines to remove wastes that might set off or maintain allergic reactions.

BACKACHE
(*see also* ARTHRITIS, KIDNEY DISORDERS, MENSTRUAL DISCOMFORT)

Backache is one of the most common physical complaints. It can be caused by injury, poor posture, muscle strain, pinched nerves, stress, or other conditions.

THE NECK — Neck problems often come from stress, holding the head in an improper position (such as looking down at a desk) for a prolonged length of time, or from injuries such as whiplash.

1. The Solar Plexus and Diaphragm Reflexes (fourteen times each, left and right sides) set up a regular breathing pattern and cause the body to relax tense muscles by stimulating the solar plexus and diaphragm.
2. The Arm and Shoulder Reflexes (fourteen times each, left and right sides) stimulate the shoulder, elbow, wrist, and other joints, increasing their blood circulation and relaxing the muscles around them.
3. The Spine Reflexes (fourteen times each, left and right sides) trigger the spine to enhance its flexibility and induce the spinal cord to improve its nervous responses.

THE MIDDLE AND LOWER BACK — Many middle- and lower-back problems are caused by injuries, poor posture, standing or sitting for long periods of time, tension, and improper lifting. Women often suffer backaches caused by pregnancy and menstrual problems, while men may suffer backaches from prostate problems.

1. The Solar Plexus and Diaphragm Reflexes (fourteen times each, left and right sides) prompt the solar plexus and diaphragm to set up a

regular breathing pattern and help the body relax tense abdominal muscles.

2. The Kidney Reflexes (fourteen times each, left and right sides) stimulate the kidneys to regulate their waste-elimination functions, thereby decreasing pressure on the lower back.
3. The Spine Reflexes (fourteen times each, left and right sides) encourage the spine to enhance its flexibility and to relieve strain on the sacroiliac by relaxing nearby muscles.
4. The Hip, Thigh, and Leg Reflexes (fourteen times each, left and right sides) stimulate the lower limbs, toning-up their muscles and nerves and increasing blood circulation through the joints.
5. The Sciatic Nerve Reflexes (fourteen times each, left and right sides) soothe the nerves that regulate the muscles used in standing and walking.

BLADDER DISORDERS
(see also KIDNEY DISORDERS — STONES;
MALE DISORDERS — PROSTATE DISORDERS)

The most common bladder disorders are infections, blockage, and poor sphincter control due to muscular weakness. The reflex areas listed here work to prevent infection by encouraging the urinary system to perform properly.

INFECTION — Infection of the bladder can take many forms and is usually due to the presence of germs in the kidneys, ureters, or bloodstream. Acute cystitis, the most common bladder infection, is often due to improper sanitary habits and can usually be prevented in females by wiping backward, not forward, after a bowel movement. Bladder infections will frequently show up when stress levels are high and resistance levels low.

1. The Solar Plexus and Diaphragm Reflexes (fourteen times each, left and right sides) stimulate the solar plexus to help the body to relax and fight stress.
2. The Spleen Reflex (fourteen times, left side only) stirs the spleen to perform specific infection-fighting functions.
4. The Liver Reflex (fourteen times, right side only) stimulates the liver to produce many types of antibodies while filtering out wastes.
5. The Adrenal Gland Reflexes (fourteen times each, left and right sides) stimulate these glands to regulate kidney functions and to release hydrocortisone, which fights inflammation.
6. The Kidney Reflexes (fourteen times each, left and right sides) speed the purification of the blood by stimulating the kidneys to process toxic wastes.

7. The Bladder Reflexes (fourteen times each, left and right sides) prompt the bladder to increase its blood circulation, bringing infection-fighting agents.
8. The Lymphatic System Reflexes (fourteen times each, left and right sides) trigger the lymphatic system to mobilize infection-fighting cells in the body.

INCONTINENCE — The inability to control the discharge of urine can be caused by injury, weak sphincter muscles, pressure on the bladder due to advanced pregnancy, and emotional stress.

1. The Solar Plexus and Diaphragm Reflexes (fourteen times each, left and right sides) trigger the solar plexus to send signals that help the body relax and overcome attacks of anxiety.
2. The Bladder Reflexes (fourteen times each, left and right sides) induce the bladder to regularly flush itself out, exercising and strengthening the sphincter muscles in the process.
3. (For men): The Prostate Reflexes (fourteen times each, left and right sides) stimulate this gland to keep it healthy and nonenlarged, so that it does not put pressure on the bladder or urethra.

BREASTS
(see FEMALE DISORDERS, MENSTRUAL DISCOMFORT)

BRONCHITIS

This inflammation of the lining of the bronchial tubes is usually caused by a bacterial or viral infection. Bronchitis often appears when the body's resistance is lowered, frequently as a complication from a cold.

1. The Solar Plexus and Diaphragm Reflexes (fourteen times each, left and right sides) trigger the solar plexus and diaphragm to help the lungs in their breathing functions.
2. The Lung Reflexes (fourteen times each, left and right sides) stimulate the lungs and bronchial tubes to fight inflammation and constriction.
3. The Adrenal Gland Reflexes (fourteen times each, left and right sides) prompt these glands to secrete hydrocortisone to reduce tissue inflammation, and epinephrine (Adrenalin) to open up the air passages.
4. The Lymphatic System Reflexes (fourteen times each, left and right sides) stimulate the lymph glands to mobilize disease-fighting cells in the body.

BURSITIS

Bursitis is a painful inflammation of the fluid-filled sac, known as the bursa, which cushions a joint against friction when it moves. The elbows, shoulders, knees, hips, and ankles can all be affected by bursitis.

1. The Adrenal Gland Reflexes (fourteen times each, left and right sides) stimulate the adrenal glands, which trigger the secretion of hydrocortisone, a natural form of cortisone that reduces tissue inflammation.
2. The Kidney Reflexes (fourteen times each, left and right sides) prompt the kidneys to process wastes out of the body in order to prevent them from collecting around the joints.
3. The Arm and Shoulder Reflexes (fourteen times each, left and right sides) and/or the Hip, Thigh, and Leg Reflexes (fourteen times each, left and right sides) stimulate the joints and limbs, increasing their blood circulation and removing the wastes that have built up around them.

COLITIS AND DIVERTICULITIS
(see also INDIGESTION)

These painful abdominal conditions are inflammations of the lining of the large intestine or colon.

1. The Adrenal Gland Reflexes (fourteen times each, left and right sides) stimulate these glands to secrete norepinephrine, to maintain intestinal muscle tone, and hydrocortisone, to reduce tissue inflammation.
2. The Intestine Reflexes (fourteen times each, left and right sides) stimulate the small and large intestines to contract regularly and remove wastes.
3. The Lymphatic System Reflexes (fourteen times each, left and right sides) stimulate the lymph glands to mobilize disease-fighting cells in the body, raising its resistance to infection.

COMMON COLD
(see also BRONCHITIS, SINUSITIS)

This well-known infection is due to a wide variety of viruses. Its symptoms include nasal congestion, sneezing, runny eyes, muscle aches, coughing, and occasional fever.

1. The Pituitary Gland Reflexes (fourteen times each, left and right sides) stimulate the gland to secrete the hormones that trigger the functions of all the other glands in the body.
2. The Sinus Reflexes (fourteen times each, left and right sides) trigger the sinuses to drain accumulated debris and to fight inflammation of their mucous membranes.
3. The Ear Reflexes (fourteen times each, left and right sides) stimulate the ears to increase their blood circulation, speeding removal of any infectious matter.
4. The Lung Reflexes (fourteen times each, left and right sides) encourage the lungs and bronchial tubes to fight constriction, increasing the oxygen levels in the blood.
5. The Adrenal Gland Reflexes (fourteen times each, left and right sides) prompt these glands to secrete epinephrine (Adrenalin), which opens up the air passages.
6. The Lymphatic System Reflexes (fourteen times each, left and right sides) stimulate the lymphatic system to fight infections throughout the body.

CONSTIPATION
(see also FLATULENCE, INDIGESTION)

Constipation is the term that is used to describe difficult or sluggish bowel movements. These are often accompanied by gas and abdominal discomfort and caused by improper diet, stress, absence of convenient toilet facilities, or dehydration.

1. The Solar Plexus and Diaphragm Reflexes (fourteen times each, left and right sides) stimulate the solar plexus to send metabolic instructions to the abdominal organs.
2. The Stomach Reflexes (fourteen times each, left and right sides) prompt the stomach to efficiently perform its food-mashing functions.
3. The Pancreas Reflexes (fourteen times each, left and right sides) induce the pancreas to secrete important digestive juices.
4. The Liver Reflex (fourteen times, right side only) triggers the liver to secrete bile to aid in proper digestion.
5. The Gallbladder Reflex (fourteen times, right side only) stimulates the gallbladder to release bile into the intestines, which acts as a mild laxative.
6. The Adrenal Gland Reflexes (fourteen times each, left and right sides) stimulate these glands to secrete hormones that enhance the muscle tone of the digestive organs.
7. The Intestine Reflexes (fourteen times each, left and right sides) prompt the small and large intestines to contract regularly to remove wastes.

DEPRESSION
(see STRESS)

DIZZINESS
(see EAR DISORDERS, HIGH BLOOD PRESSURE, NAUSEA)

EAR DISORDERS

The ears are subject to many disorders. The outer ear is vulnerable to bacterial and fungal infections, as well as cuts, burns, frostbite, and ruptured eardrums from direct blows or sudden loud noises. Middle-ear problems are usually the result of upper-respiratory infections from viruses and bacteria. The inner ear is affected by allergies, infections, and reactions to certain medications. Inner-ear problems may result in vertigo, nausea, tinnitus, and temporary or permanent deafness.

DEAFNESS — Deafness is a partial or total loss of hearing. When it is permanent — caused by disease, injury, or birth defects — it is untreatable. If it is temporary — due to blockage by ear wax or foreign objects, reactions to certain drugs, exposure to loud sounds, or severe emotional stress — it is often treatable or sometimes likely to disappear on its own.

1. The Solar Plexus and Diaphragm Reflexes (fourteen times each, left and right sides) trigger the solar plexus to send signals that help the body relax and overcome feelings of anxiety.
2. The Ear Reflexes (fourteen times each, left and right sides) trigger the ears to increase their blood circulation, stimulating the aural nerves.
3. The Arm and Shoulder Reflexes (fourteen times each, left and right sides) prompt the shoulders and arms to relax their muscles, decreasing tension in the upper torso.
4. The Spine Reflexes (fourteen times each, left and right sides) trigger the spinal cord to send relaxation signals to surrounding muscles, particularly the neck muscles.

DIZZINESS — The sensation of whirling or light-headedness is usually associated with a loss of balance. Dizziness may be caused by infections in the inner ear, sudden movements, reactions to certain drugs, and nervous disorders that affect the motions of the liquid in the inner ear's semicircular canals, which control the body's equilibrium.

1. The Brain Reflexes (fourteen times each, left and right sides) stimulate the brain to send signals that regulate the nervous system and the body's sense of equilibrium.

2. The Sinus Reflexes (fourteen times each, left and right sides) encourage the sinuses to drain accumulated debris.
3. The Ear Reflexes (fourteen times each, left and right sides) stimulate the ears to function efficiently in controlling the body's sense of balance.
4. The Eye Reflexes (fourteen times each, left and right sides) trigger the eyes to perform their seeing functions properly, fighting vertigo and distortion.

INFECTION — Infection of the ear is very common in young children, usually as an offshoot of respiratory-tract infections. Other causes are bacterial and fungal infections that enter the outer ear from water or other foreign matter.

1. The Ear Reflexes (fourteen times each, left and right sides) trigger the ears to increase their blood circulation in order to expel infectious matter.
2. The Spleen Reflex (fourteen times, left side only) stimulates the spleen to release specific antibodies to fight infection.
3. The Liver Reflex (fourteen times, right side only) induces the liver to perform its waste-filtering and infection-fighting functions.
4. The Lymphatic System Reflexes (fourteen times each, left and right sides) stimulate the lymphatic system to remove toxic wastes and to release antibodies to fight infections.

TINNITUS — A ringing, hissing, or buzzing in the ears that has no external origin is known as tinnitus. The causes of tinnitus are many and varied and not completely understood. Tinnitus can be triggered emotionally, brought on by reactions to drugs, or it can come as a result of actual physical damage to nerves in the ear.

1. The Solar Plexus and Diaphragm Reflexes (fourteen times each, left and right sides) stimulate the solar plexus to send signals that help overcome stress reactions and attacks of anxiety.
2. The Sinus Reflexes (fourteen times each, left and right sides) encourage the sinuses to drain accumulated debris.
3. The Ear Reflexes (fourteen times each, left and right sides) trigger the ears and aural nerves to function properly by increasing their blood circulation.

EYE DISORDERS

There are many types of eye disorders, some permanent, and some temporary and thus treatable. The most common temporary eye problems are due to surface injuries, infections, weakened muscles, and overuse, especially under poor lighting conditions.

EYESTRAIN — Excessive eye fatigue, or eyestrain, often results in headaches. Its causes include stress, overuse of the eyes in close work or at video or computer monitors, poor lighting, and incorrect eyeglass or contact-lens prescriptions.

1. The Solar Plexus and Diaphragm Reflexes (fourteen times each, left and right sides) prompt the solar plexus to send signals that relax the body and reduce tension.
2. The Kidney Reflexes (fourteen times each, left and right sides) trigger the kidneys to regulate fluid balances and blood pressure.
3. The Eye Reflexes (fourteen times each, left and right sides) stimulate the eyes to increase their blood and lymph circulation, refreshing tired tissues.
4. The Arm and Shoulder Reflexes (fourteen times each, left and right sides) stimulate the arms and shoulders to relax their muscles, taking the strain off the neck muscles.
5. The Spine Reflexes (fourteen times each, left and right sides) trigger the spinal cord to send relaxation signals to surrounding muscles, particularly the neck muscles.
6. The Lymphatic System Reflexes (fourteen times each, left and right sides) encourage the lymphatic system to relieve and refresh the cornea in a nutrient bath.

INFECTION — Eye infections are caused by viruses and bacteria. Some of the most common eye infections are found on the corneal surface, on the lining of the eyelid (conjunctivitis is a good example), or in the sebaceous glands, the glands that secrete skin oils, near the eyelashes (referred to as sties).

1. The Eye Reflexes (fourteen times each, left and right sides) stimulate the eyes to increase their blood and lymph circulation, removing toxic wastes and soothing irritated tissues.
2. The Spleen Reflex (fourteen times, left side only) induces the spleen to release specific antibodies to fight infection.
3. The Liver Reflex (fourteen times, right side only) stimulates the liver to perform its waste-filtering and infection-fighting functions.
4. The Kidney Reflexes (fourteen times each, left and right sides) trigger the kidneys to purify the blood and process wastes out of the body.
5. The Lymphatic System Reflexes (fourteen times each, left and right sides) trigger the lymphatic system to mobilize infection-fighting cells and to flush out the cornea, removing toxic wastes.

VISION — When problems develop in vision, a number of factors, individually or in combination, come into play. These include the shape of the eyeball, the strength of its muscles, and the health of the optic nerve and its centers in the brain.

1. The Brain Reflexes (fourteen times each, left and right sides) trigger the brain to perform and enhance its neurological functions.
2. The Eye Reflexes (fourteen times each, left and right sides) stimulate the eyes to increase their blood circulation to the optic nerves.
3. The Liver Reflex (fourteen times, right side only) triggers the liver to store and release vitamin A, necessary for good night vision.
4. The Lymphatic System Reflexes (fourteen times each, left and right sides) stimulate the lymphatic system to refresh the cornea in a nutrient bath.

FATIGUE

Feelings of chronic tiredness may be due to causes such as overwork, poor nutrition, stress, and illness.

1. The Brain Reflexes (fourteen times each, left and right sides) prompt the brain to enhance its neurological functions.
2. The Lung Reflexes (fourteen times each, left and right sides) trigger the lungs to increase the oxygen level in the blood in order to invigorate the body's tissues.
3. The Heart Reflex (fourteen times, left side only) stimulates the heart to pump oxygen-rich blood from the lungs to the brain and other organs.
4. The Liver Reflex (fourteen times, right side only) triggers the liver to release stored energy nutrients into the bloodstream.
5. The Adrenal Gland Reflexes (fourteen times each, left and right sides) induce these glands to release epinephrine (Adrenalin) to fight fatigue and speed up reaction time.

FEMALE DISORDERS
(see also BLADDER DISORDERS — INFECTION; INFERTILITY; MENSTRUAL DISCOMFORT)

The term *female disorders* is a catchall phrase used to describe those problems which are specific to females. These tend to be related to the reproductive system.

BREAST PROBLEMS — The most common breast problems in women are swelling and soreness just before menstrual periods and during pregnancy, and the constant or intermittent presence of benign cysts in the breasts.

1. The Pituitary Gland Reflexes (fourteen times each, left and right sides) stimulate the pituitary gland, which controls sexual development, milk production, and hydrocortisone production.
2. The Adrenal Gland Reflexes (fourteen times each, left and right sides) stimulate these glands to secrete hydrocortisone, reducing tissue swelling.
3. The Kidney Reflexes (fourteen times each, left and right sides) trigger the kidneys to regulate the fluid balances of the body in order to fight swelling.
4. The Ovary Reflexes (fourteen times each, left and right sides) stimulate the ovaries to regulate female-hormone secretion.
5. The Lymphatic System Reflexes (fourteen times each, left and right sides) trigger the lymphatic system to increase circulation and prevent the buildup of wastes.
6. The Breast Reflexes (fourteen times each, left and right sides) stimulate the breasts to function efficiently.

INFECTION — Infections in the female reproductive system have several sources. Germs (gonorrhea and herpes, for example) may be introduced through sexual contact with an infected partner. In addition, organisms that are naturally present (such as yeast) may sometimes grow out of proportion in numbers, due to stress, lowered resistance, or a disturbance in the body's chemical balance.

1. The Solar Plexus and Diaphragm Reflexes (fourteen times each, left and right sides) help to fight stress by triggering the solar plexus to send signals that help the body relax.
2. The Spleen Reflex (fourteen times, left side only) triggers the spleen to release specific antibodies to fight infection and to filter out impurities in lymph fluid.
3. The Liver Reflex (fourteen times, right side only) stimulates the liver to perform its waste-filtering and infection-fighting functions.
4. The Kidney Reflexes (fourteen times each, left and right sides) speed the filtering of the blood by prompting the kidneys to process toxic wastes.
5. The Ovary Reflexes (fourteen times each, left and right sides) stimulate the ovaries to fight off infections by increasing their blood and lymph circulation.
6. The Lymphatic System Reflexes (fourteen times each, left and right sides) trigger the lymphatic system to mobilize infection-fighting cells and remove accumulated toxic wastes.
7. The Uterus Reflexes (fourteen times each, left and right sides) prompt the uterus to maintain healthy functions and ward off infections.

FLATULENCE

Flatulence is an uncomfortable condition due to an excess of gas in the stomach and intestines. Flatulence is caused primarily by swallowing air or eating certain gas-causing foods, such as beans.

1. The Stomach Reflexes (fourteen times each, left and right sides) encourage the stomach to perform its food-mashing functions.
2. The Liver Reflex (fourteen times, right side only) triggers the liver to secrete bile, which breaks down food into usable nutrients.
3. The Gallbladder Reflex (fourteen times, right side only) triggers the gallbladder to release the bile it has stored, which breaks down food and moves it smoothly through the intestine.
4. The Intestine Reflexes (fourteen times each, left and right sides) stimulate the small and large intestines to contract regularly in order to prevent stagnation and expel excess gas.

FORGETFULNESS

A lapse in memory is most commonly brought on by stress, a lack of attention, or exhaustion.

1. The Solar Plexus and Diaphragm Reflexes (fourteen times each, left and right sides) prompt the solar plexus to induce calmness by relaxing the abdominal muscles.
2. The Pituitary Gland Reflexes (fourteen times each, left and right sides) stimulate the gland to secrete the hormones that trigger the functions of all the other glands in the body.
3. The Brain Reflexes (fourteen times each, left and right sides) stimulate the brain to enhance its neurological functions.
4. The Thyroid and Parathyroid Gland Reflexes (fourteen times each, left and right sides) encourage these glands to regulate muscle tension and metabolic rates.
5. The Adrenal Gland Reflexes (fourteen times each, left and right sides) induce these glands to release epinephrine (Adrenalin), triggering alertness.

GALLSTONES

Gallstones are solid particles that can range in size from microscopic crystals to rocks the size of limes. They precipitate out of bile that has become too concentrated in the gallbladder.

1. The Liver Reflex (fourteen times, right side only) stimulates the liver to manufacture fresh bile to replace and flush out over-concentrated bile in the gallbladder.

2. The Gallbladder Reflex (fourteen times, right side only) triggers the gallbladder to flush itself out regularly.
3. The Intestine Reflexes (fourteen times each, left and right sides) stimulate the small and large intestines to trigger bile release from the gallbladder and to pass stones out of the body.

GOUT

This inflammation of one or more joints, especially those of the big toe, comes from an excess of uric acid in the blood, perhaps due to hormonal imbalances that affect the functions of the kidneys.

1. The Pituitary Gland Reflexes (fourteen times each, left and right sides) stimulate the gland to secrete the hormones that coordinate the functions of all the other glands in the body.
2. The Spleen Reflex (fourteen times, left side only) triggers the spleen to regulate uric-acid production.
3. The Adrenal Gland Reflexes (fourteen times each, left and right sides) induce these glands to release hydrocortisone, which fights inflammation.
4. The Kidney Reflexes (fourteen times each, left and right sides) trigger the kidneys to regulate their uric-acid production and to process wastes out of the body that might otherwise collect at the joints.

HAY FEVER

Hay fever is a noncontagious allergic response to substances in the air, such as pollen and pollution. The symptoms of hay fever are usually seasonal and include inflamed eyes, sinuses, and nasal passages, with an occasional sore throat and irritated bronchial tubes.

1. The Solar Plexus and Diaphragm Reflexes (fourteen times each, left and right sides) trigger the solar plexus and diaphragm to help the lungs in their breathing functions.
2. The Pituitary Gland Reflexes (fourteen times each, left and right sides) stimulate the gland to secrete hormones that control the functions of all the other glands in the body.
3. The Lung Reflexes (fourteen times each, left and right sides) encourage the lungs and bronchial tubes to perform without constriction.
4. The Adrenal Gland Reflexes (fourteen times each, left and right sides) trigger these glands to secrete epinephrine (Adrenalin) to open up the air passages, and hydrocortisone, the natural form of cortisone, to reduce tissue inflammation.

HEADACHE

(see also EYE DISORDERS, EAR DISORDERS, MIGRAINE)

Painful sensations within the head or across the forehead are due to a number of causes. Some of the most common are toxic reactions to alcohol or drugs, food allergies or poor diet, tension in neck and shoulder muscles, vision problems, excessive noise or glaring light, and emotional stress.

1. The Solar Plexus and Diaphragm Reflexes (fourteen times each, left and right sides) trigger the solar plexus to send signals that help the body relax, fight stress, and overcome attacks of anxiety.
2. The Brain Reflexes (fourteen times each, left and right sides) stimulate the brain to regulate and enhance its neurological functions.
3. The Sinus Reflexes (fourteen times each, left and right sides) trigger the sinuses to flush out accumulated debris that builds up internal pressure.
4. The Ear Reflexes (fourteen times each, left and right sides) stimulate the ears to increase their blood circulation, removing infectious wastes and soothing damaged tissues.
5. The Eye Reflexes (fourteen times each, left and right sides) prompt the eyes to flush their tissues, soothing them and removing irritants.
6. The Pancreas Reflexes (fourteen times each, left and right sides) prompt the pancreas to regulate blood-sugar levels in the body.
7. The Arm and Shoulder Reflexes (fourteen times each, left and right sides) trigger these parts to relax muscle tension.
8. The Spine Reflexes (fourteen times each, left and right sides) prompt the spinal cord to send signals to surrounding muscles to relax.

HEART DISORDERS

The inability of the heart to perform its pumping functions smoothly can be caused by stress or high blood pressure, both of which trigger a variety of symptoms. Other disorders are arrhythmia, an irregular heart beat; plaque, a buildup of fatty blockages on arterial walls; and angina, a pain in the chest caused by lack of oxygen in the heart's tissues. The diagnosis of heart disorders should be left to professionals, but the best way to prevent most common heart disorders is by controlling stress, eating a low-fat, high-fiber diet, and exercising regularly.

1. The Solar Plexus and Diaphragm Reflexes (fourteen times each, left and right sides) trigger the solar plexus to send signals that help the body relax and overcome stress and attacks of anxiety.

2. The Thyroid and Parathyroid Gland Reflexes (fourteen times each, left and right sides) stimulate these glands to regulate the body's metabolic and pulse rates while controlling the calcium levels that are responsible for heart contractions.
3. The Lung Reflexes (fourteen times each, left and right sides) stimulate the lungs to exchange toxic carbon dioxide in the blood for the oxygen necessary for efficient metabolic reactions.
4. The Heart Reflex (fourteen times, left side only) stimulates the heart's cardiovascular action, which pumps blood throughout the body.
5. The Adrenal Gland Reflexes (fourteen times each, left and right sides) trigger the adrenals to secrete hormones that enhance the muscle tone of the heart and influence blood pressure and heartbeat by controlling sodium and potassium levels.
6. The Kidney Reflexes (fourteen times each, left and right sides) encourage the kidneys to filter out wastes from the blood and regulate the fluid balances that affect blood pressure.

HEARTBURN
(*see also* INDIGESTION)

A burning sensation in the stomach and lower esophagus is known as heartburn. It is commonly caused when the upper valve of the stomach does not close completely or relaxes accidentally. This allows gastric juices, such as hydrochloric acid, to leak up into the esophagus and irritate its lining. Heartburn can be brought on by eating too quickly or eating an unusually large meal.

1. The Solar Plexus and Diaphragm Reflexes (fourteen times each, left and right sides) trigger the solar plexus to regulate the functions of all the abdominal organs.
2. The Stomach Reflexes (fourteen times each, left and right sides) stimulate the stomach to perform its functions efficiently and encourage its sphincters to operate properly.

HEMORRHOIDS

Hemorrhoids, varicose veins of the rectum and anus, are now believed to be the inevitable result of walking upright. They are considered harmless, unless infection is present or they rupture, but they can be quite painful. Hemorrhoids, also known as piles, can be aggravated by constipation, pregnancy, and the repeated use of strong laxatives.

1. The Pancreas Reflexes (fourteen times each, left and right sides) induce the pancreas to secrete necessary digestive juices to break down foods.

2. The Liver Reflex (fourteen times, right side only) triggers the liver to secrete bile to aid in proper digestion, lessening the chances of constipation.
3. The Gallbladder Reflex (fourteen times, right side only) stimulates the gallbladder to release bile, which acts as a mild laxative.
4. The Adrenal Gland Reflexes (fourteen times each, left and right sides) stimulate these glands to secrete hormones that enhance the muscle tone of the digestive organs.
5. The Intestine Reflexes (fourteen times each, left and right sides) prompt the small and large intestines to contract regularly in order to remove wastes and prevent constipation.

HIGH BLOOD PRESSURE

High blood pressure is a condition in which the heart is forced to pump harder to provide proper circulatory functions. High blood pressure has a variety of causes, including hereditary predisposition, obesity, stress, diseases of the heart, kidney disorders, and disturbances in the functions of the glands, particularly the pituitary, thyroid, and parathyroid glands. Some of the symptoms of high blood pressure are dizziness, nausea, and headaches.

1. The Solar Plexus and Diaphragm Reflexes (fourteen times each, left and right sides) trigger the solar plexus to send signals that help the body combat stress and attacks of anxiety.
2. The Pituitary Gland Reflexes (fourteen times each, left and right sides) stimulate the gland to secrete hormones that regulate the functions of all the other glands in the body.
3. The Thyroid and Parathyroid Gland Reflexes (fourteen times each, left and right sides) trigger the glands to monitor the body's metabolic and pulse rates while regulating the calcium levels that are responsible for heart contractions.
4. The Heart Reflex (fourteen times, left side only) stimulates the heart's cardiovascular functions that pump blood throughout the body.
5. The Adrenal Gland Reflexes (fourteen times each, left and right sides) trigger these glands to secrete hormones that enhance the muscle tone of the heart and control the sodium and potassium levels that influence the body's blood pressure.
6. The Kidney Reflexes (fourteen times each, left and right sides) encourage the kidneys to filter out wastes from the blood and to regulate the fluid balances that affect blood pressure.

IMPOTENCE
(*see* MALE DISORDERS)

INDIGESTION
(see also HEARTBURN, NAUSEA)

Indigestion is a general term for abdominal discomfort during or just after eating. It is often caused by stress, depression, or the improper functioning of one or more of the organs in the digestive system.

1. The Solar Plexus and Diaphragm Reflexes (fourteen times each, left and right sides) trigger the solar plexus to signal the nerves and organs in the abdomen to relax.
2. The Stomach Reflexes (fourteen times each, left and right sides) prompt the stomach to perform its food-mashing functions efficiently.
3. The Pancreas Reflexes (fourteen times each, left and right sides) stimulate the pancreas to release digestive juices to break down food thoroughly.
4. The Liver Reflex (fourteen times, right side only) triggers the liver to process nutrients and to remove wastes and irritants.
5. The Gallbladder Reflex (fourteen times, right side only) triggers the gallbladder to release its stored bile to emulsify fats and act as a mild laxative.
6. The Intestine Reflexes (fourteen times each, left and right sides) stimulate the intestines to regulate their digestive and excretory functions.

INFERTILITY

Infertility is the inability to reproduce. Its causes are many and include blocked fallopian tubes or testicles (often remedied surgically), poor sperm production, hormonal imbalances, and emotional stress, among others.

1. The Solar Plexus and Diaphragm Reflexes (fourteen times each, left and right sides) trigger the solar plexus to fight stress by sending soothing, relaxing signals to the body.
2. The Pituitary Gland Reflexes (fourteen times each, left and right sides) stimulate this gland to secrete the hormones that orchestrate the functions of all the other glands.
3. The Ovary and Testicle Reflexes (fourteen times each, left and right sides) spark these glands to secrete sex hormones and reproductive cells.
4. The Uterus and Prostate Reflexes (fourteen times each, left and right sides) encourage the good health of these organs by increasing their blood circulation and enhancing their protective functions for sperm and eggs.

INSOMNIA
(*see* SLEEP DISORDERS)

KIDNEY DISORDERS
(*see also* BLADDER DISORDERS)

The inability of the kidneys to perform their waste-removal and water-balancing functions smoothly is due to a variety of causes, including stress, infection, and high blood pressure. Some of the common kidney disorders are nephritis, an inflammation of the kidneys; pyelitis, an infection of the part of the kidney known as the pelvis; kidney stones, solid particles that precipitate out of fluid wastes; and uremia, the complete failure of the kidneys.

INFECTION — Kidney infections have many causes, including bacteria and toxic materials in the blood. If left medically untreated, kidney infections may result in uremia and eventual death.

1. The Spleen Reflex (fourteen times, left side only) stimulates the spleen to release antibodies.
2. The Adrenal Gland Reflexes (fourteen times each, left and right sides) prompt these glands to encourage the kidneys to flush out by regulating fluid balances in the body.
3. The Kidney Reflexes (fourteen times each, left and right sides) stimulate the kidneys to increase their blood-circulation and waste-elimination processes.
4. The Bladder, Ureter, and Urethra Reflexes (fourteen times each, left and right sides) induce the bladder to regularly flush itself out, flushing the ureters and urethra in the process.
5. The Lymphatic System Reflexes (fourteen times each, left and right sides) stimulate the lymph glands to secrete antibodies that fight infection.

NEPHRITIS — This inflammation of the kidneys can be acute (triggered by scarlet fever or other streptococcus-caused diseases) or chronic (developing over a period of time and due to causes such as infections or reactions to drugs or toxic materials).

1. The Pituitary Gland Reflexes (fourteen times each, left and right sides) stimulate the pituitary to secrete hormones that manage the amount of urine that flows out of the body.
2. The Spleen Reflex (fourteen times, left side only) triggers the spleen to release infection-fighting antibodies.
3. The Adrenal Gland Reflexes (fourteen times each, left and right sides) prompt these glands to release hydrocortisone to fight tissue inflammation.

4. The Kidney Reflexes (fourteen times each, left and right sides) stimulate the kidneys to increase their blood circulation and to flush themselves out.
5. The Bladder, Ureter, and Urethra Reflexes (fourteen times each, left and right sides) induce these body parts to regularly flush toxic wastes out of the body.
6. The Lymphatic System Reflexes (fourteen times each, left and right sides) stimulate the lymph glands to mobilize the necessary antibodies to fight infection.

STONES — These particles precipitate out of the fluids that filter through the kidneys. While the chemistry of kidney stones varies, the most common are formed from calcium salts or excessive uric acid that has crystallized. Kidney stones can be very painful, especially if they become lodged in the ureters or the urethra as they are being passed out of the body. They can block the flow of urine, producing dangerous, even life-threatening, complications.

1. The Pituitary Gland Reflexes (fourteen times each, left and right sides) trigger this gland to release hormones that determine how much urine flows out of the body.
2. The Thyroid and Parathyroid Gland Reflexes (fourteen times each, left and right sides) prompt these glands to regulate calcium and phosphorus levels in the body.
3. The Spleen Reflex (fourteen times, left side only) prompts the spleen to regulate uric-acid production
4. The Adrenal Gland Reflexes (fourteen times each, left and right sides) trigger the adrenals to secrete anti-inflammants and to control sodium and potassium levels.
5. The Kidney Reflexes (fourteen times each, left and right sides) stimulate the kidneys to regulate their filtering functions and to flush themselves out.
6. The Bladder, Ureter, and Urethra Reflexes (fourteen times each, left and right sides) induce the bladder to regularly flush itself out, passing stones out of the body.
7. The Lymphatic System Reflexes (fourteen times each, left and right sides) stimulate the lymph glands to secrete antibodies that fight infection.

LEG CRAMPS

This painful condition is caused by sudden and involuntary tightening of the muscles of the lower limbs, especially the calf muscles. Its causes include nutritional deficiencies, fatigue, strain, or tight clothing that restricts circulation.

1. The Thyroid and Parathyroid Gland Reflexes (fourteen times each, left and right sides) stimulate these glands to regulate muscle tension.
2. The Hip, Thigh, and Leg Reflexes (fourteen times each, left and right sides) trigger these areas to increase their blood circulation and relax their muscles.
3. The Sciatic Nerve Reflexes (fourteen times each, left and right sides) trigger the sciatic nerve to send relaxation signals to lower-limb muscles.

LIVER DISORDERS

The inability of the liver to perform its wide-ranging functions smoothly can have a variety of causes, including infections, exposure to toxic substances, and obstructions. Early warning signs of liver trouble include jaundice — yellowish skin and eyes from too much bile in the blood — abnormal stools, and, in severe cases, vomiting blood.

CIRRHOSIS — This degeneration of the cells of the liver, with their replacement by fibrous scar tissue, results in obstructed blood flow in the liver and disruption of the liver's vital functions. Cirrhosis can be induced by repeated exposures to toxins and alcohol, hepatitis, certain forms of cardiovascular disease, or poor diet. If caught in its early stages, cirrhosis can be treated medically and nutritionally.

1. The Thyroid and Parathyroid Gland Reflexes (fourteen times each, left and right sides) trigger these glands to regulate the body's metabolic rates.
2. The Liver Reflex (fourteen times, right side only) stimulates the liver to increase its blood circulation and heal damaged tissue.
3. The Gallbladder Reflex (fourteen times, right side only) prompts the gallbladder to regulate the amount of bile it stores and releases.
4. The Kidney Reflexes (fourteen times each, left and right sides) stimulate the kidneys to flush toxic wastes out of the body.

HEPATITIS — This inflammation of the liver comes from a number of causes that include viral and bacterial infections, improperly sterilized syringes, and contaminated blood transfusions, as well as from exposure to toxic substances such as arsenic, alcohol, poisonous mushrooms, and carbon tetrachloride.

1. The Spleen Reflex (fourteen times, left side only) triggers the spleen to perform its lymph-filtering and infection-fighting functions.

2. The Liver Reflex (fourteen times, right side only) stimulates the liver to release antibodies to fight infection and increase its blood circulation, flushing out toxic wastes.
3. The Gallbladder Reflex (fourteen times, right side only) encourages the gallbladder to regulate the amounts of bile that it releases.
4. The Lymphatic System Reflexes (fourteen times each, left and right sides) set the lymphatic system in motion to fight infection and raise the body's resistance to disease.

LUNG DISORDERS
(*see also* ASTHMA, BRONCHITIS)

The inability of the lungs to perform their breathing functions may be caused by infections, inflammation, abscesses, and emphysema.

1. The Solar Plexus and Diaphragm Reflexes (fourteen times each, left and right sides) stimulate these parts of the body to regulate the actions of the lungs.
2. The Lung Reflexes (fourteen times each, left and right sides) trigger the lungs to perform their breathing functions and heal their damaged tissues.
3. The Adrenal Gland Reflexes (fourteen times each, left and right sides) stimulate the adrenals to release hydrocortisone to fight inflammation and epinephrine (Adrenalin) to alleviate closed air passages.

MALE DISORDERS
(*see also* BLADDER DISORDERS, INFERTILITY)

The catchall term *male disorders* is used to describe those problems which are specific to males and are generally related to reproductive processes.

IMPOTENCE — The temporary or permanent inability to achieve or maintain an erection. Impotence strikes almost every man at some point, usually due to exhaustion, emotional stress, or excessive intake of alcohol and certain drugs. Other causes of impotence are many and include diabetes, syphilis, and other diseases.

1. The Solar Plexus and Diaphragm Reflexes (fourteen times each, left and right sides) trigger the solar plexus to send relaxing signals to abdominal areas, relieving stress.
2. The Pituitary Gland Reflexes (fourteen times each, left and right sides) stimulate the pituitary gland to release hormones that regulate all glandular functions in the body.

3. The Brain Reflexes (fourteen times each, left and right sides) invigorate the brain so that it properly regulates physical and emotional reactions.
4. The Thyroid and Parathyroid Gland Reflexes (fourteen times each, left and right sides) induce these glands to regulate the calcium levels in the body that control muscle tension.
5. The Testicle Reflexes (fourteen times each, left and right sides) stimulate the testicles to regulate their male-hormone secretions.
6. The Prostate Reflexes (fourteen times each, left and right sides) trigger the prostate to increase its blood circulation, enhancing its health.

PROSTATE DISORDERS — The most common prostate disorders are prostatitis, the inflammation of the prostate due to infections such as gonorrhea, and benign enlargement, perhaps related to hormonal changes and common in men after the age of fifty. Cancer of the prostate is one of the most common forms of malignancy in men over the age of sixty-five.

1. The Pituitary Gland Reflexes (fourteen times each, left and right sides) stimulate the pituitary to secrete the hormones that regulate all the glandular functions in the body.
2. The Spine Reflexes (fourteen times each, left and right sides) encourage the spinal cord to align the body's nervous responses and relax the muscles around the spine and sacroiliac.
3. The Testicle Reflexes (fourteen times each, left and right sides) stimulate the testicles to perform their reproductive functions and secrete testosterone, the male sex hormone that regulates male sexual functions.
4. The Lymphatic System Reflexes (fourteen times each, left and right sides) prompt the lymph nodes to increase their infection-fighting abilities.
5. The Prostate Reflexes (fourteen times each, left and right sides) stimulate the prostate to fight infections and to secrete the alkaline fluid needed to transport and protect sperm.

MENOPAUSE

Menopause is the span of time in a woman's life when her menstrual cycles diminish and eventually stop, ending her childbearing abilities. During menopause the ovaries slow or stop their estrogen production. Some of the problems women suffer during menopause include hot flashes, sudden weight gain or loss, insomnia, heart palpitations, and the loss of bone calcium due to hormonal changes.

1. The Pituitary Gland Reflexes (fourteen times each, left and right sides) stimulate the pituitary to regulate all glandular functions in the body.
2. The Brain Reflexes (fourteen times each, left and right sides) trigger the brain to control the physical and emotional activities of the body.
3. The Thyroid and Parathyroid Gland Reflexes (fourteen times each, left and right sides) stimulate these glands to regulate calcium and phosphorus levels in the body to prevent bone-calcium loss.
4. The Ovary Reflexes (fourteen times each, left and right sides) stimulate the ovaries to regulate their estrogen secretion to fightbone-calcium loss and many of the unpleasant effects of menopause.
5. The Uterus Reflexes (fourteen times each, left and right sides) encourage the uterus to maintain its health and flexibility, even though its childbearing functions are over.

MENSTRUAL DISCOMFORT
(*see also* ANEMIA; BACKACHE — MIDDLE AND LOWER BACK)

There are a number of symptoms that are related to menstrual cycles. These include premenstrual tension, painful menses, water retention, swollen breasts, and backache.

BREAST SORENESS — This painful condition that causes the breasts to retain excess fluid and swell is due to the hormonal changes that are part of the menstrual cycle.

1. The Pituitary Gland Reflexes (fourteen times each, left and right sides) trigger the pituitary to secrete ACTH, the adrenal-stimulating hormone that controls the adrenal glands' release of anti-inflammants.
2. The Adrenal Gland Reflexes (fourteen times each, left and right sides) stimulate these glands to respond to ACTH stimulation and release hydrocortisone to reduce swelling in the breasts.
3. The Kidney Reflexes (fourteen times each, left and right sides) prompt the kidneys to perform their water-level regulation in the body to prevent tissue swelling.
4. The Breast Reflexes (fourteen times each, left and right sides) stimulate the breasts to increase their blood and lymph circulation to remove wastes and excess fluids.
5. The Ovary Reflexes (fourteen times each, left and right sides) stimulate the ovaries to regulate their secretion of female sex hormones.

CRAMPS — Cramps are caused by the sudden contraction of the uterus and surrounding abdominal, back, and thigh muscles. There are many causes of menstrual cramps. They include poor nutrition, lack of calcium, a narrow or bent cervix, stress, and exhaustion.

1. The Solar Plexus and Diaphragm Reflexes (fourteen times each, left and right sides) stimulate the solar plexus to regulate tension levels in the body by signaling the abdominal muscles to relax.
2. The Thyroid and Parathyroid Gland Reflexes (fourteen times each, left and right sides) stimulate these glands to maintain proper blood-calcium levels.
3. The Spine Reflexes (fourteen times each, left and right sides) prompt the spine and spinal cord to relax the areas around them, relieving tension.
4. The Uterus Reflexes (fourteen times each, left and right sides) stimulate the uterus to maintain its elasticity and to efficiently perform its monthly flushing functions.

PREMENSTRUAL TENSION — There are many uncomfortable symptoms related to menstrual cycles. These include weight gain due to fluid retention, emotional irritability, and depression. Premenstrual tension is believed to be caused by the disorderly secretion of certain hormones, such as progesterone.

1. The Pituitary Gland Reflexes (fourteen times each, left and right sides) regulate the pituitary, which sends out hormones that control all the body's glandular functions.
2. The Brain Reflexes (fourteen times each, left and right sides) stimulate the brain to perform its regulatory functions and fight emotional stress.
3. The Thyroid and Parathyroid Gland Reflexes (fourteen times each, left and right sides) stimulate these glands to maintain blood-calcium levels that determine the body's level of tranquility.
4. The Adrenal Gland Reflexes (fourteen times each, left and right sides) trigger these glands to fight bloating and swelling by releasing hydrocortisone, an anti-inflammant.
5. The Kidney Reflexes (fourteen times each, left and right sides) stimulate the kidneys to flush out excess fluids from the body and to maintain water balance in the tissues.
6. The Ovary Reflexes (fourteen times each, left and right sides) stimulate the ovaries to regulate the secretion levels of their female hormones, especially progesterone.
7. The Uterus Reflexes (fourteen times each, left and right sides) encourage the uterus to stay healthy and discharge, without problem, its lining and the unfertilized egg.

MIGRAINE

A migraine is a severe form of headache that usually affects only one side of the head. It is often preceded by flashes of light, a spot, or a flickering in the center of the field of vision, and is sometimes accompanied by nausea and dizziness. Causes of migraine are still unknown, but it is believed to be triggered by disturbances in blood circulation in the brain. Stress, exhaustion, glandular imbalances, allergies, and cardiovascular problems such as high blood pressure may be contributing factors.

1. The Solar Plexus and Diaphragm Reflexes (fourteen times each, left and right sides) trigger the solar plexus to send signals that overcome feelings of anxiety and stress.
2. The Pituitary Gland Reflexes (fourteen times each, left and right sides) stimulate the gland to secrete the hormones that regulate the functions of all the other glands in the body.
3. The Brain Reflexes (fourteen times each, left and right sides) stimulate the brain to regulate organic functions and to fight emotional stress.
4. The Heart Reflex (fourteen times, left side only) stimulates the heart's cardiovascular action, which pumps blood throughout the body.
5. The Adrenal Gland Reflexes (fourteen times each, left and right sides) influence blood pressure by triggering the adrenal glands to regulate sodium and potassium levels.
6. The Kidney Reflexes (fourteen times each, left and right sides) encourage the kidneys to filter wastes from the blood and to regulate fluid balances that affect blood pressure.

MOTION SICKNESS
(*see* EAR DISORDERS, NAUSEA)

NAUSEA
(*see also* EAR DISORDERS, INDIGESTION)

Nausea is the unpleasant sensation that often precedes vomiting. The causes of nausea are innumerable and include digestive problems, stress, balance problems, and infectious diseases such as influenza.

1. The Solar Plexus and Diaphragm Reflexes (fourteen times each, left and right sides) trigger the solar plexus to send signals that help the body fight stress and prompt the diaphragm to enhance breathing operations to increase oxygen levels in the body.

2. The Brain Reflexes (fourteen times each, left and right sides) stimulate the brain to control equilibrium and fight emotional stress.
3. The Ear Reflexes (fourteen times each, left and right sides) stimulate the ears to control the body's sense of balance by regulating the fluids in the semicircular canals.
4. The Stomach Reflexes (fourteen times each, left and right sides) prompt the stomach to relax and normalize its food mashing functions.
5. The Intestine Reflexes (fourteen times each, left and right sides) stimulate the small and large intestines to contract regularly to prevent stagnation and the backflow of wastes.

PHLEBITIS

Phlebitis is the inflammation of a vein, particularly a vein in the leg. It is usually caused by a clot that has formed in the vein due to slow circulation or injury.

1. The Heart Reflex (fourteen times, left side only) stimulates the heart to perform the cardiovascular action that keeps blood pumping smoothly throughout the body.
2. The Liver Reflex (fourteen times, right side only) triggers the liver to regulate blood-clotting functions in the body.
3. The Adrenal Gland Reflexes (fourteen times each, left and right sides) stimulate the adrenal glands to release hormones that enhance the muscle tone of the heart and reduce inflammation.

PREGNANCY
(*see* BACKACHE; BLADDER DISORDERS — INCONTINENCE;
FEMALE DISORDERS; INFERTILITY; MENSTRUAL DISCOMFORT)

PROSTATE DISORDERS
(*see* MALE DISORDERS)

SCIATICA

Also known as sciatic neuritis, sciatica is an inflammation of the sciatic nerves due to injury, constipation, cold temperatures, and arthritis, among other causes.

1. The Adrenal Gland Reflexes (fourteen times each, left and right sides) trigger these glands to secrete a natural anti-inflammant known as hydrocortisone.

2. The Intestine Reflexes (fourteen times each, left and right sides) stimulate the small and large intestines to contract regularly to prevent constipation.
3. The Spine Reflexes (fourteen times each, left and right sides) prompt the spinal cord to send relaxing signals to surrounding muscles, especially those near the sacroiliac.
4. The Hip, Thigh, and Leg Reflexes (fourteen times each, left and right sides) stimulate the lower limbs to increase their circulation and relax muscles.
5. The Sciatic Nerve Reflexes (fourteen times each, left and right sides) stimulate the sciatic nerves to soothe their responses and to resist inflammation.

SHINGLES

Shingles are a painful viral infection of a nerve ending, often triggered by stress and sometimes accompanied by blisters. The shingles virus, herpes zoster, is the same one that causes chicken pox.

1. The Solar Plexus and Diaphragm Reflexes (fourteen times each, left and right sides) trigger the solar plexus to send signals that help the body relax and fight stress.
2. The Spine Reflexes (fourteen times each, left and right sides) prompt the spinal cord to soothe the body's nervous responses and to relax the muscles around the spine.
3. The Lymphatic System Reflexes (fourteen times each, left and right sides) stimulate the lymphatic system to increase the body's resistance to disease.

SINUSITIS

Sinusitis is an inflammation of the mucous membranes that line the sinuses. Frequently, sinusitis triggers the sinuses to fill with pus. Some of its causes are allergies, exposure to pollutants, exposure to temperature extremes, and upper respiratory-tract infections.

1. The Pituitary Gland Reflexes (fourteen times each, left and right sides) stimulate the pituitary to regulate the functions of all the other glands in the body.
2. The Sinus Reflexes (fourteen times each, left and right sides) trigger the sinuses to drain any debris that has accumulated in them and to fight infection and inflammation of their mucous membranes.

3. The Adrenal Gland Reflexes (fourteen times each, left and right sides) trigger these glands to release hydrocortisone, to fight inflammation, and epinephrine (Adrenalin), to open clogged breathing passages.
4. The Lymphatic System Reflexes (fourteen times each, left and right sides) stimulate the lymphatic system to prevent toxic-waste buildup in the body and to release antibodies to fight infections.

SKIN DISORDERS

There are a great number of disorders of the skin. These include: dry skin — from poor nutrition, harsh chemicals, dehydration, and glandular imbalances; oily skin — from a diet rich in fatty foods and from glandular imbalances; acne — from glandular imbalances, improper diet, and infection; and rashes — from allergies and stress.

1. The Pituitary Gland Reflexes (fourteen times each, left and right sides) stimulate the gland to secrete the hormones that balance all the glandular functions in the body.
2. The Thyroid and Parathyroid Gland Reflexes (fourteen times each, left and right sides) stimulate these glands to regulate metabolic rates in the body.
3. The Liver Reflex (fourteen times, right side only) triggers the liver to store and release vitamin A for balanced skin oil, to regulate nutrient absorption, and to release antibodies to fight infections.
4. The Adrenal Gland Reflexes (fourteen times each, left and right sides) trigger the adrenal glands to regulate the metabolism of fats, proteins, and carbohydrates, as well as to fight inflammation of sebaceous glands and ducts.
5. The Kidney Reflexes (fourteen times each, left and right sides) encourage the kidneys to filter out toxic substances from the blood and to regulate the water balances in the tissues.
6. The Ovary and Testicle Reflexes (fourteen times each, left and right sides) trigger these reproductive glands to regulate their hormonal secretions.
7. The Lymphatic System Reflexes (fourteen times each, left and right sides) stimulate the lymphatic system to remove toxic wastes from the body and to release antibodies to fight skin infections.

SLEEP DISORDERS
(see also STRESS)

The inability to sleep is due to several factors, including emotional stress, excitement, high blood pressure, and a number of illnesses or neurological disorders.

1. The Solar Plexus and Diaphragm Reflexes (fourteen times each, left and right sides) trigger the solar plexus to send signals that help the body relax, fight panic reactions, and overcome feelings of anxiety.
2. The Brain Reflexes (fourteen times each, left and right sides) stimulate the brain to regulate the functions of the hypothalamus, which controls sleep patterns.
3. The Thyroid and Parathyroid Gland Reflexes (fourteen times each, left and right sides) stimulate these glands to regulate calcium levels in the body to keep muscles relaxed.
4. The Spine Reflexes (fourteen times each, left and right sides) prompt the spinal cord to soothe the body's nervous responses and to relax the muscles around the spine.

STRESS

Stress is a state of tension that manifests itself as anxiety, fear, or depression. A number of factors cause stress, such as the loss of a family member, a move, a change in job, financial worries, and divorce.

1. The Solar Plexus and Diaphragm Reflexes (fourteen times each, left and right sides) prompt the solar plexus to signal the abdominal muscles and organs to relax.
2. The Pituitary Gland Reflexes (fourteen times each, left and right sides) trigger the gland to align specific hormonal balances in the body, bringing about a calming sensation.
3. The Thyroid and Parathyroid Gland Reflexes (fourteen times each, left and right sides) prompt these glands to bring muscle tension into balance, which affects the overall tranquility of the body.
4. The Lung Reflexes (fourteen times each, left and right sides) stimulate the lungs to increase the blood's oxygen level, thus inducing metabolic processes that refresh and nurture the body.
5. The Kidney Reflexes (fourteen times each, left and right sides) encourage the kidneys to align the fluid balances that affect blood pressure, while removing irritating toxic wastes from the body.
6. The Spine Reflexes (fourteen times each, left and right sides) encourage the spinal cord to signal the muscles around the spine to relax.

ULCERS

An ulcer is an open sore that is not a wound, but is inflamed and slow to heal. The most common ulcers are peptic ulcers, areas of erosion on the mucous lining of the stomach, esophagus, and intestine.

Exactly what triggers digestive ulcers is still not known, but stress seems to play a major role.

1. The Solar Plexus and Diaphragm Reflexes (fourteen times each, left and right sides) trigger the solar plexus to send signals that help the body overcome feelings of tension and anxiety.
2. The Stomach Reflexes (fourteen times each, left and right sides) stimulate the stomach to increase blood circulation to its tissues, bringing necessary healing agents.
3. The Adrenal Gland Reflexes (fourteen times each, left and right sides) stimulate the adrenal glands to control blood pressure and to secrete hydrocortisone to fight tissue inflammation.
4. The Intestine Reflexes (fourteen times each, left and right sides) motivate the small and large intestines to contract regularly to prevent their contents from stagnating by staying in one place.

VARICOSE VEINS
(see also HEMORRHOIDS, PHLEBITIS)

Distended, swollen veins, usually visible just below the surface of the skin on the legs, are known as varicose veins. Varicose veins often appear knotted and make the legs feel fatigued, sore, and prone to cramps and swelling. Varicose veins are probably the result of standing upright and can be aggravated by long periods of standing or sitting in one position.

1. The Heart Reflex (fourteen times, left side only) stimulates the heart to pump blood smoothly throughout the body.
2. The Adrenal Gland Reflexes (fourteen times each, left and right sides) trigger the adrenals to release hormones that enhance the muscle tone of the heart and to regulate blood pressure by controlling sodium and potassium levels.
3. The Hip, Thigh, and Leg Reflexes (fourteen times each, left and right sides) stimulate the lower limbs to increase their blood circulation to prevent clotting and relieve swelling.

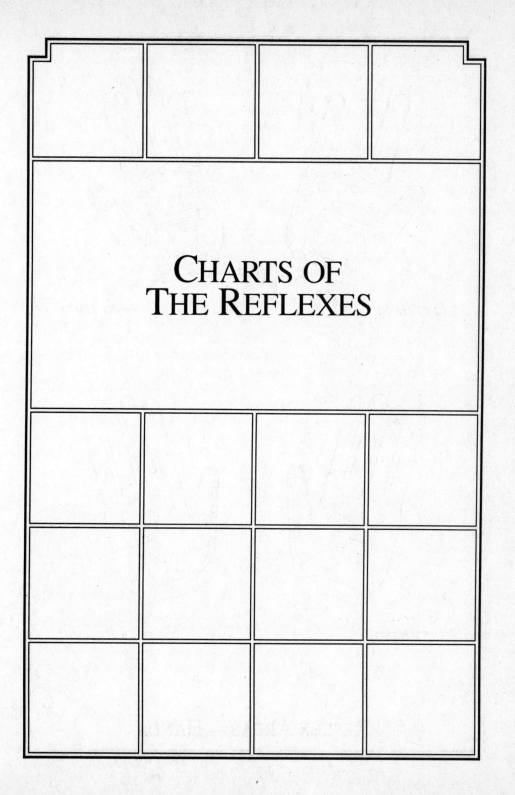

CHARTS OF
THE REFLEXES

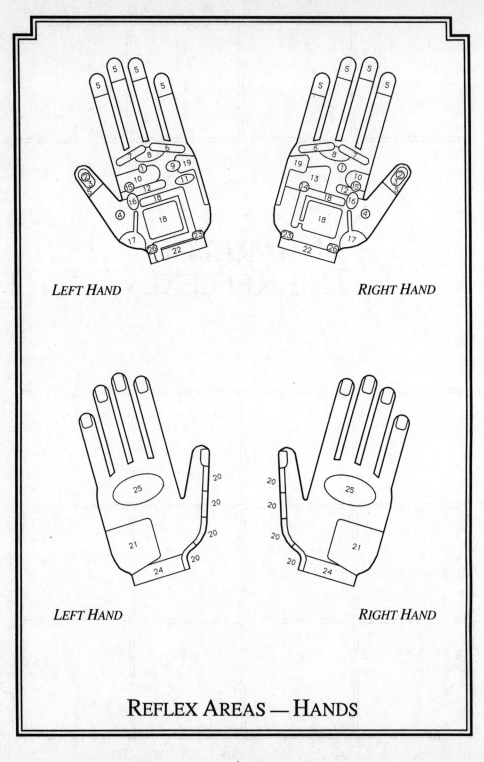

LEFT HAND

RIGHT HAND

LEFT HAND

RIGHT HAND

REFLEX AREAS — HANDS

REFLEX AREAS — HANDS

1. The Solar Plexus and Diaphragm Reflexes (both hands).
2. The Pituitary Gland Reflexes (both hands).
3. The Brain Reflexes (both hands).
4. The Thyroid and Parathyroid Gland Reflexes (both hands).
5. The Sinus Reflexes (both hands).
6. The Ear Reflexes (both hands).
7. The Eye Reflexes (both hands).
8. The Lung Reflexes (both hands).
9. The Heart Reflex (left hand only).
10. The Stomach Reflexes (both hands).
11. The Spleen Reflex (left hand only).
12. The Pancreas Reflexes (both hands).
13. The Liver Reflex (right hand only).
14. The Gallbladder Reflex (right hand only).
15. The Adrenal Gland Reflexes (both hands).
16. The Kidney Reflexes (both hands).
17. The Bladder, Ureter, and Urethra Reflexes (both hands).
18. The Intestine Reflexes (both hands).
19. The Arm and Shoulder Reflexes (both hands).
20. The Spine Reflexes (both hands).
21. The Hip, Thigh, and Leg Reflexes (both hands).
22. The Sciatic Nerve Reflexes (both hands).
23. The Ovary and Testicle Reflexes (both hands).
24. The Lymphatic System Reflexes (both hands).
25. The Breast Reflexes (both hands).
26. The Uterus and Prostate Reflexes (both hands).

LEFT FOOT

RIGHT FOOT

BOTH FEET

REFLEX AREAS — FEET

REFLEX AREAS — FEET

1. The Solar Plexus and Diaphragm Reflexes (both feet).
2. The Pituitary Gland Reflexes (both feet).
3. The Brain Reflexes (both feet).
4. The Thyroid and Parathyroid Gland Reflexes (both feet).
5. The Sinus Reflexes (both feet).
6. The Ear Reflexes (both feet).
7. The Eye Reflexes (both feet).
8. The Lung Reflexes (both feet).
9. The Heart Reflex (left foot only).
10. The Stomach Reflexes (both feet).
11. The Spleen Reflex (left foot only).
12. The Pancreas Reflexes (both feet).
13. The Liver Reflex (right foot only).
14. The Gallbladder Reflex (right foot only).
15. The Adrenal Gland Reflexes (both feet).
16. The Kidney Reflexes (both feet).
17. The Bladder, Ureter, and Urethra Reflexes (both feet).
18. The Intestine Reflexes (both feet).
19. The Arm and Shoulder Reflexes (both feet).
20. The Spine Reflexes (both feet).
21. The Hip, Thigh, and Leg Reflexes (both feet).
22. The Sciatic Nerve Reflexes (both feet).
23. The Ovary and Testicle Reflexes (both feet).
24. The Lymphatic System Reflexes (both feet).
25. The Breast Reflexes (both feet).
26. The Uterus and Prostate Reflexes (both feet).